EVERYBODY'S GUIDE TO NATURAL SLEEP

Also by Philip Goldberg:

The Babinski Reflex
The Intuitive Edge
Executive Health

Also by Daniel Kaufman:

The One Day at a Time Diet
Ireland: Presences
How to Get Out of Debt without Despair
  and without a Lawyer

EVERYBODY'S GUIDE TO
NATURAL SLEEP

*A Drug-Free Approach to Overcoming
Insomnia and Other Sleep Disorders*

PHILIP GOLDBERG
and
DANIEL KAUFMAN

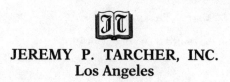

JEREMY P. TARCHER, INC.
Los Angeles

To our wives, Jane and Gina—and to
the Kaufmans' daughter, Anastasia—
whose love makes it possible for the
respective authors to sleep in peace.

Library of Congress Cataloging in Publication Data

Goldberg, Philip, 1944–
    Everybody's guide to natural sleep / Philip Goldberg and Daniel
Kaufman.
        p.   cm.
    Rev. ed. of: Natural sleep. c1978.
    Includes bibliographical references.
    1. Insomnia—Popular works.   I. Kaufman, Daniel.   II. Goldberg,
Philip, 1944–   Natural sleep.   III. Title.
    RC548.G63   1990
        616.8'498—dc20   90-31407
        ISBN 0-87477-570-1   CIP

Copyright © 1990 by Philip Goldberg and Daniel Kaufman

Jeremy P. Tarcher, Inc.
5858 Wilshire Blvd., Suite 200
Los Angeles, CA 90036

Distributed by St. Martin's Press, New York

Manufactured in the United States of America
10 9 8 7 6 5 4 3 2 1

First Edition

Contents

A flock of sheep that leisurely pass by,
One after one; the sound of rain, and bees
murmuring; the fall of rivers, winds and seas,
Smooth fields, white sheets of water, and pure sky,
I have thought of all by turns and yet do lie
Sleepless! . . .
Come, blessed barrier between day and day
Dear mother of fresh thoughts and joyous health!

WILLIAM WORDSWORTH

How many thousand of my poorest subjects
Are at this hour asleep!
O sleep, O gentle sleep,
Nature's soft nurse, how have I frighted thee,
That thou no more wilt weigh my eyelids down
And steep my sense in forgetfulness?

SHAKESPEARE, *Henry IV, Part II*

Acknowledgments

We would like to express our gratitude to the many professionals who so generously shared their knowledge with us as we prepared both the original and revised editions: Dr. Harold Bloomfield, Samuel Bursuk, David Cohen, Dr. Allan Cott, Norman Dine, Dr. Joe D. Goldstrich, Dr. Mark Goulston, Dr. Peter Hauri, Dr. Ernest Hartmann, Dr. Oscar Janiger, Dr. German Nine-Murcia, Dr. Elliot Phillips, Dr. Charles Pollack, Dr. Quentin Regestein, Dr. Brian Rees, Elizabeth Sandler, Dr. Jon Sassin, Dr. Art Spielman, Dr. Michael Stevenson, Ron Teeguarden, Dr. Michael Thorpy, and Dr. Elliot Weitzman.

In addition, we deeply appreciate the advice, support, and patience that we received from our families and friends, especially during the long and often tedious process of compiling information for the original edition.

Finally, we are specially indebted to the many insomniacs who shared their experiences with us. May this book put them all safely to sleep.

Foreword

*T*his is a well-written and amazingly complete do-it-yourself guide to the treatment of insomnia. I think that basically it does an excellent job.

As a scientist and a physician involved in the field of sleep, I approached the request to write a Foreword with some hesitancy. As a scientist, I was afraid that a book written by reporters for the general public might be so full of inaccuracies, or shortcuts to avoid difficult terminology, as to make it misleading. However, this does not turn out to be the case. The scientific inaccuracies here are small and are not of great importance. They do not interfere with the general meaning or flow of the book.

As a physician, of course, my concern was that such a book might lead people to try dangerous treatments or might lead them to avoid proven medical treatments for specific medical conditions. Again, I feel the authors have basically done a good job. They are aware that insomnia has many causes, and that some of these causes involve treatable medical and psychiatric illness, and the authors are careful to suggest in many places that consultation with a physician or with a sleep clinic may be required. There is perhaps one place where I would add a caution in addition to those provided by the authors: a sudden and drastic change in diet can sometimes be dangerous, especially in a person who has liver disease or kidney disease or is taking various medications. The authors rightly warn of the dangers of taking drugs such as sleeping pills, which can disrupt the delicate machinery of the body in many ways. Unfortunately, such disruption can sometimes also be caused by the sudden addition or withdrawal of natural food substances as well as by the addition of substances labeled as medications.

In its listing and discussion of do-it-yourself treatments for insomnia, this book is breathtakingly complete. It discusses the use of foods, diets, bedtime rituals, exercise, massage, breathing techniques, relaxation, hypnosis, herbal remedies, regularity of habits, and even such things as types of sheets, blankets, and bedrooms. All this makes fascinating reading for the good sleeper as well as the insomniac, and I learned a number of things I had not known before. I am slightly disturbed by the shotgun approach in which hundreds of possible remedies are suggested to the reader, with fairly well-established and scientifically based treatments handled in more or less the same way as really "far out" and unlikely forms of help. However, I must admit that even the most "far out" and illogical-sounding approach has probably sometimes helped someone to sleep, and I suppose we must trust the good sense of the reader to pick and choose what appears probable to him or her from the amazing wealth of possibilities presented.

I agree strongly with the authors' stand that most sleeping pills are dangerous substances and have been overused. My own position is that clearly insomnia is not an illness for which a sleeping pill is a cure (though it has too frequently been misinterpreted in this sense). Insomnia is a symptom of many underlying conditions, and the insomniac or his physician should attempt to determine the underlying cause of the insomnia and to treat that cause. Most often the cause will be behavioral-psychological, psychiatric (anxiety or depression), or medical, and the treatment will either involve no medication, or will involve medication aimed at a specific medical or psychiatric condition, rather than a sleeping pill. There is a place for the use of sleeping pills, but it is a fairly limited place; even for this limited role, I believe we have not developed drugs in the right way. Sleeping pills so far have been nonspecific central nervous system depressants that have little to do with the physiology of sleep. I have recently done a great deal of research work, mentioned by the authors of this book, on a more "natural" substance that is not a nervous system depressant but is related to the physiology of sleep. This is a natural food substance, the amino acid l-tryptophan. I discuss my views of sleep, insomnia, and sleeping pills in my book *The Sleeping Pill*.

Overall, I believe *Everybody's Guide to Natural Sleep* may be of help to a number of persons suffering from mild or moderate insomnia who will find in it something directly useful to them. In addition, this book is fun to read.

ERNEST HARTMANN, M.D.
Director, Sleep Disorders Center,
Newton-Wellesley Hospital
Professor of Psychiatry,
Tufts University School of Medicine

Preface

*T*his is an updated version of a book that was originally published in 1978. We decided to revise and republish the work because, in the intervening years, a number of advances have been made in our understanding of sleep, and a variety of new treatments have appeared that might provide relief for many insomniacs. Although several other books with the same goals have been published since ours was first released, we felt there was still a need for our approach: to provide all the facts plus an eclectic, comprehensive selection of natural remedies for sleep problems. Despite scientific progress, there has barely been a dent in the total number of insomniacs; each one cured has been replaced by a new body tossing and turning into the long, dark night.

The main purpose of this book is to help people sleep. We have included all sensible, nondrug procedures, both orthodox and unorthodox, to give insomniacs the widest possible choice of pathways for finding natural sleep. In gathering material we relied on interviews, library research, personal observations, and both scientific and anecdotal evidence. At the same time, we did not shy away from old wives' tales, folk remedies, serendipitous discoveries, common sense, and even hunches. In many cases, we were personally unconvinced about the efficacy of a particular treatment but included it anyway—as long as it was deemed harmless—if it was taken seriously by experts or held any promise for even a small number of readers.

None of the instructions in this book should be construed as a prescription for insomnia. Neither Daniel Kaufman, who conceived this project and did most of the research, nor Philip Goldberg, who organized the material and wrote the final copy, is a medical doctor. We approached our work as journalists, attempting to be as objective as possible. Serious sleep disorders and questions of a medical nature should be taken to a physician.

There is no one cure for insomnia. We leave it to you to determine for yourself which of the natural procedures might be efficacious. The self-evaluating questionnaires and charts will help you make intelligent personal choices. You should also receive insight and guidance from the detailed discussions of sleep, insomnia, and related topics. Those sections are up-to-date and reflect the current state of scientific knowledge.

In the years since the first edition was published, the number of sleep disorder centers in the United States has gone from 6 to over 100, and there are a few hundred more in the works. This means that medical expertise about sleep is much more accessible, and research results are increasingly fed into the pipeline of knowledge. Another change has been the widespread discrediting of sleeping pills as a method of treatment. The number of prescriptions written and over-the-counter sleep-aids purchased have dropped precipitously. At the same time, the growth of the holistic health movement and the increased acceptance of alternative modalities such as acupuncture have introduced new and valuable remedies to the marketplace. All these changes are reflected in this revised edition.

Also new is the special section on children and sleep. It provides basic guidelines for helping your child establish regular, healthy sleep patterns, and for dealing with anxiety-related insomnia. Even kids can't get to sleep sometimes.

For all that is new, much remains the same as it was in 1978. There are still millions of people who can't fall asleep or stay asleep. A sleeping pill is still a cure that is worse than the disease. There is still a lot we don't know about sleep and insomnia. And you can still find something simple and natural between the covers of this book that will bring you relief under the covers of your bed.

Los Angeles, May 1990

CHAPTER 1

Your Bedtime Story

*N*ature evolves in regular, pulsating rhythms. From tiny atoms to huge clusters of galaxies, each unit of creation vibrates in cyclical fashion—up-down, in-out, stop-go. Within our bodies are over one hundred different cycles whose regular patterns affect the metabolism of our cells, the pumping of our blood, our intake of oxygen, and even our moods and states of consciousness. When these cycles mesh appropriately with one another and with the rhythms of their environments, our well-being and progress are assured, for we are then functioning as nature intended. When the rhythms are out of synchrony, as in an orchestra, cacophony results. Our bodies suffer.

The periodicity of these syncopated biological rhythms ranges from a fraction of a second to a number of years. Some, like the sleep/wake cycle that is the concern of this book, are called *circadian*, from the Latin *circa* ("approximately") and *dies* ("day"). These cycles obey the daily pattern set down by the rotation of the earth, taking approximately 24 hours to run their course.

Evening falls and flowers fold their petals. Plants fold their leaves. With the exception of owls and other nighttime predators, the creatures of land, sea, and air curl up into bedroom niches in the rocks, trees, and sand. Dawn comes and the unfolding begins. The outside world, which had been barred from the senses of the sleepers, is once again admitted.

This rhythm is the most natural thing in the world, intended no doubt to be accomplished effortlessly. Yet, an enormous number of people find themselves alarmingly disconnected from the natural flow of sleeping and waking that nature intended us to follow.

How many people suffer from insomnia? The estimates vary, ranging from 20 million to 70 million Americans, from one tenth to one third of the population. Even if we accept the most conservative estimate, that's a lot of tossing and turning. And those estimates are usually based on the number of *serious* insomniacs, the definition of which varies considerably. Some doctors define insomniacs as those who can't sleep at all; others are willing to categorize as insomniacs all those who merely complain about their sleep. The currently accepted definition, sure to become known as DIMS, is: one who has "difficulty initiating or maintaining sleep."

Several surveys have tried to pin down the exact incidence of sleep problems. Of 1,000 households surveyed in Los Angeles, one third had someone with current problems, and in 42 percent someone had suffered from sleep problems at some time. *Esquire* magazine described a Gallup poll in which 50 percent of those interviewed had trouble falling asleep or staying asleep. In Gainesville, Florida, psychiatrist Ismet Karacan surveyed 1,645 people and found that one third to one half had trouble sleeping. A University of California survey indicated that one third of the population had recurrent bouts with insomnia, and 15 percent suffered it chronically.

Polls of doctors have also been revealing, though somewhat disparate. In one survey, roughly 19 percent of the patients seen by the 3,000 doctors queried had complaints of insomnia (see accompanying table). That figure may actually understate the case, for some say that more people in the

United States visit doctors for help in getting to sleep than for any other single complaint. It is also estimated that half of those not considered insomniacs have a sleepless night on occasion, and a large but undetermined number do not sleep as efficiently as they should.

DOCTORS ESTIMATE INSOMNIA INCIDENCE AMONG PATIENTS*

Type of Practice	Incidence of Insomnia (%)
Family practice	12.8
Gastroenterology and cardiovascular disease	18.3
General practice	14.0
Internal medicine	17.5
Neurology	14.1
Obstetrics and gynecology	11.6
Pediatrics	15.5
Psychiatry	33.2
Surgery	16.4
Child psychiatry	18.6
Average	18.7

*Responses from 3,000 physicians to survey by Dr. Anthony Kales.

Insomniacs can take comfort in knowing that they are in excellent company, even if it does feel lonely in that dark room. As you roll over again and again, count sheep, make lists, or play word games; as you try to still your mind; as you contemplate what a lousy day tomorrow will be if you don't fall asleep immediately; as you inch dangerously closer to the medicine chest—you might be accompanied by as many as 50 million of your compatriots. That's a veritable epidemic.

You are also part of an ancient tradition. Although we have no way of knowing how prevalent the affliction has been in the past, the legends and lore of nearly every known culture bewail the torment of those unable to sleep. The evidence suggests that magical potions, herbs, esoteric rituals, and incantations specifically designed to induce sleep have been used for thousands of years. The tombs of ancient pharaohs, wherein all things considered indispensable for the living were lodged, are said to have contained urns of sleep-promoting herbs such as chamomile, lest the spirit of the departed monarch suffer a sleepless night. Ancient Egyptian hieroglyphs record a lament for three living hells, one of which is "to be in bed and sleep not."

From our own Western heritage, the present-day insomniac can claim as restless bedfellow the Roman poet Horace, who coined the phrase "I cannot sleep a wink" over two thousand years ago. Proust, Kafka, Kipling, Nietzsche, and Poe are but a few of the notables whose writings record bouts with sleeplessness. The irrepressible Mark Twain has supplied us with enough quips on the subject to enable us to laugh our way to sleep. And so many of Shakespeare's characters lyrically toss and turn across the pages of his plays that one twentieth-century pedant was moved to write a book titled *Shakespeare's Insomnia.*

Those starved for what Shakespeare called the "chief nourisher of life's feast" come in three basic categories. The most prevalent are those who can't fall asleep on going to bed and who remain awake for what usually seems an eternity, even though they feel exhausted mentally and physically. Clinicians term this type of sleep disorder *initial* insomnia.

The second type was well described by Franz Kafka: "I fall asleep soundly, but after an hour I wake up, as though I had laid my head in the wrong hole. I . . . have before me anew the labour of falling asleep and feel myself rejected by sleep." Called *intermittent* insomnia, this type of sleep disorder may recur any number of times in a given night and seems more prevalent among the middle-aged and elderly, especially those with physical disorders.

In the third category—*matutinal* or *terminal* insomnia—are those who fall asleep well enough but wake up prematurely, usually after five or six hours, dull, weary, unrefreshed, and unable to fall back to sleep.

Some authorities add a category for those who simply do not sleep well. That is, they fall asleep fairly promptly, awaken after a reasonable length of time, say, seven or eight hours, but are not as refreshed as they should be and are fatigued during the day. Their sleep is *inefficient*. That category might include many people (perhaps a large majority) who would never think of calling themselves insomniacs.

There is reasonable evidence to suggest that we are, as a nation, chronically deprived of proper sleep.

With the advent of electric lights, human beings began to break from the rest of nature, engaging in stimulating activity later and later into the night. Television and other entertainment opportunities further aggravated this new pattern. Yet, unlike our ancestors who typically went to sleep not long after sundown, we tend to get up when we must, not when we want to or feel a natural need to. In an article in the *Bulletin of Psychosomatic Society*, Drs. W. B. Webb and H. W. Agnew reported several studies to support the notion that we are chronically sleep-deprived: the sleep of young students surveyed in 1910 and 1911 was 1½ hours longer than a 1963 comparison group; a more recent survey of 1,000 students revealed that a third found it "very hard to get up in the morning," and less than a third woke up refreshed and rested. Other surveys revealed that students typically slept an hour longer on weekends, and that when left on their own in a schedule-free situation, they exceeded their usual sleep by more than an hour.

If you have picked up this book for any reason other than idle curiosity, the chances are that you frequently or occasionally have difficulty sleeping. Or, you might be a reasonably good sleeper who is interested in improving the quality of your sleep or in avoiding the occasional sleepless night each of us encounters as a result of stress or unusual situations—travel, an important event, illness, excessive pressure at work, or a tragedy. Whatever your reason, we are confident that you will benefit from the practical suggestions in this book.

WHY THE BOOK WAS WRITTEN

Both authors were chronic insomniacs at one time. Like our fellow sleepless wonders, we reached for the handiest remedy—sleeping pills—when the problem first arose. We used both prescribed and over-the-counter varieties and soon suffered the mental and physical ravages typical among users and abusers of sleep medication, ravages that are described more fully later on. Subsequently, our sleep unimproved, we sought natural ways of dealing with sleeplessness and its consequences.

When we first began to seek out alternatives to drugs we discovered there was a striking need for a comprehensive compendium of natural ways to improve sleep. There was plenty of literature on sleep and insomnia, all of which counseled against the use of drugs, but it was mainly technical in nature—usually scholarly tomes explaining the current state of theoretical and scientific knowledge on the subject. There were books that offered practical suggestions for combating insomnia, but these were either out-of-date or heavily weighted toward one or another of the numerous approaches to sleep problems.

Many books were devoted exclusively to hackneyed, often banal platitudes that could be summarized by "learn to relax" or "don't worry." Good advice, but hardly practical, concrete, or comprehensive, and certainly not enough to coax a restless nervous system into the arms of "Nature's soft nurse," as Shakespeare called sleep.

We ended up consulting a wide variety of sources and experimenting with a wide variety of treatments. Our research helped us with our own sleep problems considerably. We still have our difficult nights, but they come with far less frequency and severity. We are no longer chronic insomniacs. On those infrequent occasions when we are sleepless, the knowledge we acquired researching this book enables us to deal with the problem without the usual worry and aggravation.

When we decided to write this book, we added to our own experiences all the material we could gather from copious reading and interviewing. The result is a how-to handbook that should aid everyone from the severe insomniac to the average person who simply wants to make the most of those mysterious nighttime hours. In our investigations we learned that science has only recently gotten around to the serious study of sleep and sleep disorders. But sleep research is off to a promising start. Like all new areas of inquiry, this one is filled with contradictory opinions, hopeful theories, wild speculation, and even controversy. It is moving at the same agonizingly slow pace with which sleep comes to insomniacs. Which is as it should be; the methods of science require complex, time-consuming processes of experimentation and repeated validation to ensure that that which is efficacious and accurate enters the mainstream of knowledge.

But time is not the only hindrance to science's understanding. We found that physicians—for reasons of their training and philosophical orientation—are, as a whole, resistant to the simple notion of looking to nature for guidance. Research funding seems to gravitate toward the complex and cumbersome rather than the simple and economical. Thus, sleep research has largely ignored obvious areas of importance, such as nutrition, choosing instead to experiment with elaborate technology, dubious pharmaceuticals, and abstract psychological contrivances.

Science's approach to sleep problems has been hampered by the same narrow perspective that has dominated our approach to health in general and that has made us a nation of pill-poppers. Because we still view body parts in isolation without regard to the whole person, medical science, despite its magnificent achievements, has structured its healing arts almost entirely on the treatment of specific, discrete symptoms. Only recently have we begun to consider the complex and delicate interaction of body, mind, spirit, and environment. Hence, insomnia has been treated, for the most part, with sleeping pills.

Now that the deleterious effects of sleep-drugs have become inescapably evident, the public has reduced its use of such medication considerably and the medical community is actively searching for alternatives. The holistic health movement, a fringe group in the seventies, moved steadily into the mainstream in the eighties. Today the idea of treating disorders such as insomnia with exercise, nutrition, psychological counseling, and even offbeat remedies such as those in this book sounds far less outrageous than it did ten or fifteen years ago. Nevertheless, reasonable alternatives to sleeping pills have not been adequately studied or reported, as medical researchers and pharmaceutical companies still put their efforts into finding one magic cure-all. However, medicine is slowly but clearly moving toward a broader, more holistic view of insomnia and of health in general.

In ancient traditional cultures the healing arts tended to view symptoms as indications of a more general malfunction of the body as a whole. Each part of the organism affects all other parts, a perspective rapidly catching on in modern medical circles. Mind, behavior, environment, and body all fit together in an organic, interconnected way to make up a unified whole that is more than a collection of the parts. Nothing can be ignored when treating any ailment.

This is especially true, we are discovering, with something as fundamental as sleep. In the case of a virus, a broken toe, or an infection, the immediate treatment of the symptom makes more sense than it does with a problem as systemic as insomnia. Insomnia is not a disease; it is a sign, or, as sleep specialists like to say, it is a *complaint*. In virtually every case, it is symptomatic of other factors—sometimes superficial and mundane, sometimes deep and serious; sometimes particular and discernible, sometimes an overall imbalance of the physiology.

One person's sleep problems may be caused by factors entirely different from those that keep the next person awake, even though the symptoms may appear to be identical. Most experts agree that sleep difficulties tend to be multifaceted. What happens when your head hits the pillow at night depends in some way on everything you did, said, felt, thought, ate, drank, and experienced from the moment you raised your head off the pillow that morning. Indeed, it is affected by every prior moment of your life. Because of this complexity, diagnosis must always be an individual matter.

In our research we tried to keep those points in mind. We tried to maintain a holistic perspective, and we urge the reader to do the same. When we turned to the experts, we discovered, to our delight, that there is a growing number of individuals—physicians, psychologists, nutritionists, and other professionals—whose perspectives are broad and whose minds are open to alternatives to conventional medicine. They are uncovering much that is useful and natural, which they have used to supplement their more orthodox training. From these persons we received a great deal of our information, and we balanced their input with standard medical opinions.

Our status as fellow sufferers enabled us to personally try out some of the methods we discuss. We also like to think it provided us with an uncommon amount of empathy. One of the problems with insomnia is that it elicits very little sympathy from others, even from friends.

"I hardly slept a wink" does not generate the same response as "I have the flu" or "I stubbed my toe." No one composes doleful tunes about sleeplessness (the Beatles' "I'm So Tired" notwithstanding), and no one will ever make a tearjerking TV movie about a nonsleeper who bravely overcomes her affliction. Insomnia is rarely even an acceptable excuse for being absent, late, forgetful, or sluggish. There aren't many outward signs—other than dark circles under your eyes—with which to elicit sympathy: no sneezes, no blood, no plaster casts to autograph, no scars to show off, no impressive Latin terms to drop. Often insomniacs encounter antipathy—even from their own spouses, who are more likely to complain about all the tossing and turning than to soothe the sleepless brow.

Most afflictions are thought of as unavoidable impositions from the outside. "Poor thing," the sufferer is told, "it could have happened to anyone." Not so with insomnia. Like an unhappy marriage or body odor, sleeplessness is usually considered self-inflicted and avoidable. Insomniacs can't file for disability if their sleep loss ends up getting them fired, nor is insomnia enough of an excuse for being bad company. No one sends insomniacs get-well cards.

Having spent a good deal of time imprisoned by insomnia, we know what it's like to go through a day with bleary eyes and rubbery knees. And we know what helped us. Therefore, this book emphasizes practical suggestions. We are convinced that insomnia can be cured naturally and easily. In most cases, you can do it yourself. "The insomniac patient should be made to understand that he or she must take charge of his own life," states sleep expert Dr. Quentin Regestein. "Don't take your body to the doctor as if he were a repair shop."

HOW TO USE THIS BOOK

The first three chapters will give you a basic understanding of the function of sleep, the causes of insomnia, and the effects of drugs. This will provide a foundation for you to properly evaluate and apply the multitude of methods available for aiding sleep. These methods, along with the guidance of your physician or psychologist when necessary, plus your own awareness of your particular needs and problems, should bring welcome relief. In many cases, complete recovery from even chronic sleeplessness will be possible. At the very least, you will be pointed in the direction of the kind of assistance you need.

The treatments and suggestions that begin in chapter 4 are divided into categories for convenience. In some cases, the category assignment is somewhat arbitrary. For example, a practice recommended for bedtime might also be employed during the day or when you are awakened during the night. In such instances, the procedure appears in the category in which it is most likely to be used, and other suggested applications are mentioned.

To make the most of the information in this book, we suggest that you underline, take notes, or in some other way annotate as you go along, marking the points that strike a familiar chord or stand out. Chances are these are the points that will be of greatest value.

Perhaps you will find that you experience certain symptoms of insomnia. Or perhaps one of the factors that causes insomnia jumps out at you from the page. Maybe some recognition will come when you are reading about some of the methods of treatment—perhaps a vitamin or a bedtime ritual strikes you as particularly interesting. These items might be engaging your attention because they have practical value for you. You are the only one who can determine which of the many methods you should try. Looking back over your notes and underlinings will give you good clues.

Since every person's sleep needs are unique, it is important to understand yourself and your own sleep patterns thoroughly. For that reason we have included charts and questionnaires for you to fill out while reading this book. We urge you to complete the forms and consider your responses carefully; you will become much more aware of your sleep problems and the factors that may be affecting them.

Some of the questionnaires can be completed as soon as you come to them; we recommend doing this before you go on to the next chapter. Other forms are meant to serve as running logs. These should be kept daily and continued for at least two weeks. The greater personal awareness the charts elicit should make your notations later in the book all the more pertinent.

When you have finished *Everybody's Guide to Natural Sleep*, go back over your charts and questionnaires. Then skim the book, paying particular attention to the sections you singled out. You will then be in a good position to judge which combination of methods will best fit your needs. Your case might call for nothing more than an eyeshade or a little more exercise. Or, you might need a radical change in diet or other habits. You might notice that you awaken at the same time every night, unable to fall back to sleep, and you may conclude that your main problem was believing you had a problem, and that a simple change of schedule does the trick. Or, you might realize that you have come to dread your bedroom because it is associated with insomnia, in which case the "stimulus control" technique in chapter 9 might be just the thing. After reading about myoclonic seizures in chapter 4, you might conclude that you need to visit a sleep specialist.

In any case, if you pay attention to your responses to the questionnaires, you are bound to end up spending more quality time in slumber and less time and money on getting there.

Solving most sleep problems requires some experimentation. Pick and choose from the potpourri of possibilities in this book. Make educated guesses. Discuss your ideas with your family, friends, and trusted health experts. Consider your budget. Be sensible and objective. And don't try so many things at the same time that you can't tell which one is having what effect. However, if you have a problem that is of major concern, don't fiddle around too long and don't spare the expense. Although it may be fickle in your case now, sleep can be one of your best friends. Treat it with respect and treat it generously.

Personal Sleep Questionnaire

This questionnaire will make you more aware of your sleep patterns, your habits, and your problems. Reference will be made to each point throughout the book.

1. Do you sleep soundly?
    Usually   Sometimes   Never

2. Do you awaken in the night?
    Usually   Sometimes   Never
    If so, how many times per night? For how long?

3. Do you ever awaken too early in the morning unable to return to sleep?
    Usually   Sometimes   Never

4. How much sleep do you get on the average night?
    Has that changed? If so, when?

5. What is your usual bedtime?
    Before 10 P.M.   Between 10 P.M. and 12 A.M.
    Between 12 and 2 A.M.   After 2 A.M.

    a. Are you usually tired at bedtime?

    b. Do you stay up long after you are sleepy?

6. What time do you usually wake up?
    Before 6 A.M.   Between 6 and 8
    Between 8 and 10   After 10 A.M.

7. Do you usually go to bed at the same time each night?

8. Do you usually get up at the same time each morning?

9. Have either your bedtime or your waking times changed recently? When? Explain the change.

10. How do you usually feel when you get out of bed in the morning?
    Alert, wide awake
    Awake, but not fully alert
    Foggy
    Still sleepy, want to sleep more

    a. Has this changed? When? Explain the change. How do you account for it?

    b. Do you use an alarm clock?

11. How long does it take you to fall asleep once you get into bed?
Less than 15 minutes
15–30 minutes
30–45 minutes
45 minutes to an hour
More than an hour

    a. Has this changed? When? Explain the change. How do you account for it?

    b. What do you think about when lying awake?

    c. What do you feel physically?

12. Do you feel that you get enough sleep?

13. When did you last fall asleep easily?

14. When did you last sleep well through the night?

15. When did you last wake up refreshed?

16. If your sleep pattern has changed, what do you think caused it?

17. How do you account for your sleep problems?

18. Do you take sleeping pills? Prescription? Over-the-counter?

    a. How often do you take them?

    b. How long have you been taking them?

19. What other medication do you take?

20. Do you drink alcohol? How much per day?

21. Do you smoke cigarettes? How many per day?

22. Do you drink coffee? How many cups per day?

23. Do you have any medical problems? What are they?

24. What do you do when you are unable to sleep at night?

25. During the day, do you ever worry about whether you will sleep that night?

26. Do you take naps during the day? How often? For how long? At what time of day?

    a. Do you often feel like napping but do not have the opportunity? At what time of day?

    b. Has this changed? When? Why?

27. Do you think that most people sleep better than you do?

28. How many hours of sleep does the average person get?

29. How much sleep do human beings need?

30. What do you think is the most common cause of insomnia?

31. Do you snore?
    Usually   Sometimes   Never

32. Does your spouse complain of being kicked in the night?
    Usually   Sometimes   Never

33. Do you have trouble breathing during your sleep?

34. Is your bedroom noisy? State the noise problem. What do you do about the noise problem?

35. Is your bedroom dark? Are you bothered by light in the morning?

36. Is the air in your bedroom too humid? too dry? too warm? too cold?

37. Do you sleep alone? If not, what size bed do you have?

38. Are your covers too heavy? too short? too binding?

39. Are you too cold at night? too warm?

40. Is your mattress comfortable? too soft? too hard?

41. What posture do you sleep in?

42. Do you bring work home with you on a regular basis?

43. How do you usually spend your last hour before going to bed?

44. Do you do anything to help you fall asleep? Bath? Relaxation technique? Foods or drinks? Exercises? Music? Other?

Stress Factors

The following is a list of life changes known to produce stress. It was compiled in 1965 by Dr. T. H. Holmes, a psychiatrist from the University of Washington, and it has been used by health experts to rate stress. The list goes from the most stressful changes to the least stressful. These stress factors often lead to disturbed sleep. Recalling which of these changes you have been exposed to may help you identify the cause of situational insomnia. Often, insomnia is precipitated by a real event and is then perpetuated for reasons discussed later on.

Which of these events has occurred in your life? For each "Yes" write how long ago it occurred and whether you noticed any change in your sleep immediately thereafter.

Event	Yes or No	Date Occurred	Sleep Change?	How?
Death of spouse				
Divorce				
Marital separation				
Jail term				
Death of close family member				
Personal injury or illness				
Marriage				
Fired at work				
Reconciled with mate				
Retirement				
Changed health in family member				
Pregnancy				
Sex difficulties				
New family member				
Business readjustment				
Changed financial status				
Death of a close friend				
Changed to a different line of work				

Event	Yes or No	Date Occurred	Sleep Change?	How?
Increased arguments with mate				
New mortgage or loan				
Foreclosure of mortgage or loan				
Changed work responsibility				
Child left home				
Trouble with in-laws				
Outstanding personal achievement				
Mate began or ended work				
Changed living conditions				
Revision of personal habits				
Trouble with boss				
Changed work hours or conditions				
Changed residence				
Changed schools				
Changed recreation				
Changed church activities				
Changed social activities				
Changed number of family meetings				
Changed eating habits				
Vacation				
Christmas				
Minor violation of law				

Diet Chart

In chapter 6, we discuss the nutritional causes of insomnia and the ways that dietary treatments can help improve sleep. To make the most of that information, we suggest that you keep the following log—it will help you to become more aware of your diet and thus make useful changes.

Every day for the next two weeks, or until you finish reading this book, keep track of everything you eat and drink.

DAY _____ **Breakfast** (note time)
Food   Drink

Snacks (note time)
Food   Drink

Lunch (note time)
Food   Drink

Snacks (note time)
Food   Drink

Supper (note time)
Food   Drink

Snacks (note time)
Food   Drink

What time did you go to bed?
At bedtime, did you feel bloated? Full? Comfortable?
    Slightly hungry? Starving? Stomach upset?
Place a * next to anything that contains caffeine
    (coffee, tea, cola, chocolate).
Place a + next to anything that contains sugar.
Plan an X next to all starchy food (breads, potatoes,
    pasta).
Place an O next to foods you salted.

Personal Sleep Record

Throughout this book we discuss many points that are relevant to people with particular sleep patterns and idiosyncrasies. This log will make you more conscious of your own.

Starting tonight, fill in this chart every day for the next two weeks, or until you finish this book, whichever is longer.

Instructions:

Mark the time you went to bed with an arrow pointing down (↓).

Mark the time you think you fell asleep with a red dot.

Mark the times you woke up (during the night or in the morning) with a green dot.

Mark the times you got out of bed with an arrow pointing up (↑).

Mark daytime naps in the same manner, or with an N.

Day	Date	10 P.M.	11 P.M.	Mid-night	1 A.M.	2 A.M.	etc.

Each day answer the following questions:

1. How long did it take you to fall asleep?

2. How many times did you wake up?

3. How much total sleep time did you get?

4. Did you have to be up at a certain time? What time?

5. Did you use an alarm clock?

6. On a scale of (a) very tired, (b) somewhat tired, (c) OK, (d) alert, (e) very alert:
   How did you feel first thing in the morning?
   How did you feel two hours after waking?
   How did you feel at lunchtime?
   How did you feel two hours after lunch?
   How did you feel at dinner time?
   How did you feel two hours after dinner?
   How did you feel at bedtime?

Psychological Factors

In chapter 7 and elsewhere in the book, we discuss the attitudes and emotional problems that contribute to insomnia. These questions will help you evaluate those factors in your own life.

1. Do you tend to worry a lot? What things worry you? Your health? Your love life or loss of love? Your financial situation or loss of money? Death? Others?

2. Do you get depressed?
   Often   Sometimes   Never

3. Do you get nervous anticipating a difficult day?

4. Are you thought of as ambitious?

5. Are you impatient?

6. Are you often restless?

7. Do you find it hard to relax?

8. Do you enjoy competition? Do you fear it?

9. Are you aggressive?

10. Are you unable to separate work from play?

11. Do you take your problems home with you? Do you take your problems to bed with you?

12. Do you drive yourself too hard?

13. Do you take time to relax?

14. Do you argue with your family? Do you argue at night?

15. Are you known as a person with a good sense of humor?

16. Do you seek the respect of others? Do you fear losing it?

17. Are you easily hurt? When was the last time someone hurt you? Explain what happened.

18. Do you get angry?
    Often   Sometimes   Seldom
    What angers you? Do you express your anger or do you hold it in?

19. Do you face your problems squarely? Do you tend to make excuses? Do you pretend things are going well when they are not?

20. Have you ever had psychiatric treatment? How long? Why did you go? Why did you stop?

21. Are you easily startled or shaken up? What causes that?

22. Do you cry easily? Do you tend to keep your sadness to yourself?

23. Do you lose your temper easily?

24. Do you respond well to pressure? or do you "go to pieces"?

25. Do you have trouble letting go and enjoying yourself?

CHAPTER 2

What Is Sleep?

Now, blessings light on him that first invented sleep! It covers a man all over, thoughts and all, like a cloak; it is meat for the hungry, drink for the thirsty, heat for the cold and cold for the hot. It is the current coin that purchases all the pleasures of the world cheap, and the balance that sets the king and the shepherd, the fool and the wise man even.

CERVANTES, *Don Quixote*

*F*ew of us can say it with the poetic grace of Cervantes, but we all need to sleep, just as we need to breathe and to eat. The reason remains a mystery to science. Why is sleep necessary? How much of it do we need? How do we fall asleep? What goes on in our bodies and minds during sleep? Why do some of us not sleep well? To obtain the answers, a growing amount of time, energy, and money is being devoted to research in sleep laboratories and clinics across the country.

By monitoring the physiological processes that occur during sleep; by studying the effects of sleep deprivation, changes in natural sleep patterns over time and differences in sleep habits among different groups of people under different conditions; and by studying the sleep of animals, researchers are uncovering a great deal of information. But they still do not have a complete, precise, irrefutable set of answers.

A report from the sleep clinic at New York's Montefiore Hospital sums up the state of the art: "Beginnings have been made in answering questions about what sleep is, what functions it serves, and of how people fall asleep, awaken, and remain awake. Despite these promising beginnings, however, virtually the whole field of sleep remains to be explored."

WHAT HAPPENS WHEN WE SLEEP?

At one time scientists believed that in sleep all bodily functions shut down completely. Not so. It turns out that sleep is a highly dynamic state, nearly as active and complex as ordinary waking consciousness. During sleep, the bodily systems follow regular, oscillating cycles, which differ only insignificantly from one person to another. Scientists have distinguished two distinct stages of sleep, each as different from the other as either is from the waking state. These are called *REM* and *non-REM* (or *NREM*). The distinctions will be clear in a moment.

When you first fall asleep, you slip into NREM sleep, which then proceeds in four discrete stages (see the following chart). In Stage I, the muscles start to relax, breathing becomes regular, body temperature begins to fall, but the sleeper, on the border of wakefulness, can be aroused easily, and might even claim not to have been asleep at all. It is a shallow stage of sleep.

During Stages II and III, sleep becomes progressively deeper. The body processes slow down still further, and it becomes more and more difficult to awaken the sleeper. In Stage IV, the deepest stage of sleep, breathing is even; heart rate, blood pressure, and body temperature are all low and fall to their lowest levels.

A NORMAL NINETY MINUTE SLEEP CYCLE	Stage	Brain Waves
	Threshold of sleep	Steady, even alpha rhythms 9–12 cycles per second.
	Stage I	Smaller, slower, pinched, irregular, variable.
	Stage II	Larger, occasional quick bursts.
	Stage III	Slow, large (5 times as big as stage I), about one per second.
	Stage IV	Very large delta waves; slow, jagged pattern.
	REM	Irregular, small, big bursts, resembles waking.

Then comes what is called the REM state, named after the *rapid eye movements* that occur just as though the sleeper were watching a moving picture. This is the state in which most dreaming occurs, and has, in fact, become synonymous with the dream state. The bodily processes change more radically—the sleeper is limp, the chin muscles are slack, but blood pressure, heart rate, and respiratory rate, all of which had lowered during the four NREM stages, elevate, becoming more variable. The brain-wave patterns, which had gradually become larger, smoother, and slower, now begin to resemble the active, irregular patterns of the waking state.

The evidence indicates that a higher level of mental and nervous-system activity goes on during REM. It had once been thought that the rapid eye movements and the penile erections that occur at that time were reactions to the contents of dreams. This has since been refuted. "It is now realized," states a publication from Montefiore's clinic, "that rapid

Behavior and experiences	Depth of sleep	Bodily activity
Relaxation, mind wanders, awareness dull.	Borderline.	Slowing down, muscular tension decreasing.
Drifting thoughts and dreams, floating feeling.	Easily awakened, might deny having slept.	Gradual slowing down, pulse growing more even, breathing more regular, temperature falling.
Some thought-like fragments; eyes will not see if opened.	Easily awakened by sounds.	Continued decrease of all bodily functions (blood pressure, metabolism, secretions, pulse, etc.), eyes may roll slowly from side to side.
More removed from outer world, rarely able to recall thoughts or dreams.	More difficult to awaken—takes louder noise.	All processes continue to drop.
Virtual oblivion, poor recall; a rare nightmare; if a sleep walker or bed wetter, those begin now.	Very difficult to awaken; the deepest sleep.	Continued decrease to deepest state of physical rest.
Rapid eye movements, dreaming vividly about 85% of the time.	Difficult to bring back to reality.	Chin muscles slack; blood pressure, pulse, breath irregular; penile erections; toes and fingers may twitch.

eye movements and penile erections are caused by centers of the brain that differ from those that produce dreams. Thus caused by mental activity but goes on at the same time as the mental activity."

These cycles—beginning with NREM and ending with REM—last about 90 to 100 minutes. Four or five such cycles occur during the average night's sleep. Everyone, whether an insomniac or a normal sleeper, follows these basic patterns (NREM always precedes REM except in infants, narcoleptics, and those deprived of sleep for more than 200 hours). The differences lie in the amount of time spent in the various stages: poor sleepers tend to spend less time in the valuable Stage IV and REM states, and they also have the cycles disrupted more frequently by periods of wakefulness. With aging, the amounts of total sleep, REM sleep, and Stage III and IV sleep all decrease, an important point for elderly readers to bear in mind, and one we shall return to later on.

WHY MUST WE SLEEP AT ALL?

Theories about the reasons we sleep range from the obvious to the bizarre. One postulates that sleep first arose as a mechanism for restoration following periods of exertion. Like any machine, the theory goes, the human body needs occasional rest and maintenance, so it shuts down at regular intervals. In this view, sleep persisted in the course of evolution because it had important survival value. A related theory contends that sleep evolved as a preventive device meant to forestall fatigue during subsequent periods of exertion. Another holds that sleep did not evolve at all; it was always an important and fundamental feature of nature's orderly, rhythmic ways, as basic as eating.

Other theories are more imaginative and intriguing but a bit hard to swallow. For example, some anthropologically oriented theorists claim that sleep patterns arose because predators had nothing to do at those times of day when their prey was, for one reason or another, impossible to catch. So sleep was relegated to times when hunting would be unprofitable. This, of course, may explain *when* we sleep, but it doesn't explain *why* we sleep. A parallel theory contends that our early ancestors would have been ill-equipped to protect themselves when foraging about in the dark. Since it was in the interest of self-preservation to be cut off from stimulation during those dangerous hours, they invented sleep.

Those with a psychoanalytic bent have their ideas too. Wrote Sigmund Freud: "Somatically, sleep is an act which reproduces intrauterine existence, fulfilling the conditions of repose, warmth, and absence of stimulus"—the famous return to the womb. Although Freud did not contend that the above analysis identified the *only* reason for sleep, some of his orthodox followers have gone that far, or quite nearly so, and have stretched Freud's logic beyond reason.

Common sense tells us that sleep must be, at the very least, restorative. Yet, that simple observation has not yet been proven to the satisfaction of scientists. Says Dr. Peter Hauri, director of the Sleep Center at the Mayo Clinic in Rochester, Minnesota: "The fact is, from a strictly neurological and physiological viewpoint, there is no objective proof that any restorative or recuperative processes get under way. And yet we all know, subjectively, that sleep makes us feel better—that we feel refreshed by a good night's sleep and feel miserable when we are sleepless."

The accompanying chart represents approximations, based on a report in the *Journal of the American Medical Association*, of three different sleep patterns: a normal one, an insomniac's, and an insomniac on large doses of sleeping pills. Note that the insomniac spent more time awake, took longer to fall asleep, and spent less time in Stages III and IV and in REM. The drug user never reached Stage III or IV, and had little REM.

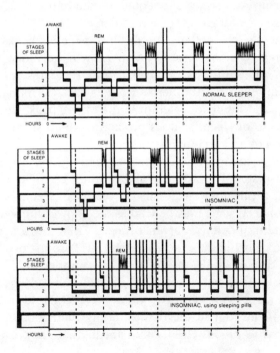

Although our experience tells us that sleep restores vigor to the body, we now know from research that it does more than merely relieve ordinary physical fatigue. Writes Dr. William C. Dement, one of the pioneer researchers on the subject: "While it is true that muscular fatigue will be ameliorated while the body is 'at rest' during the night, it seems clear that the reversal of fatigue is not the specific function of sleep or the sole reason for its existence."

The elimination of waste products, respite from emotional tension, resynthesis of brain tissue, the cathartic purging of psychic stress—all have been suggested as reasons for the obvious importance of sleep. Studies have indicated, for example, that the ongoing replacement of cells in the body intensifies during sleep. Research also bears out a common experience: good sleep makes the mind work better. In one study, children who were two or three years behind the normal rate of progress in school quickly caught up when encouraged to sleep whenever they felt fatigued.

Evidently, the activity of certain hormones peaks during deep sleep. One of these, human growth hormone (HGH), helps in the synthesis of protein and regulates the body's growth and repair. Another hormone, parathormone, which regulates the supply of calcium in the blood, peaks during the latter hours of sleep, as does prolactin, which stimulates the formation of milk in nursing mothers.

Perhaps the most exciting recent finding links sleep to the immune system. As a result of his study on rabbits, James Krueger, a physiologist at the University of Tennessee, suggests that deep sleep may be vital to the body's ability to mobilize its natural defenses against illness. Even more significant is a study on humans by University of Toronto psychiatrist Harvey Moldofsky. He found that the number of T lymphocytes (cells that help destroy abnormal cells) drops significantly during sleep. Says Dr. Moldofsky: "It could mean that the T cells are out in the tissues, doing their job, and aren't found in the blood. Or it could mean that they're inactive during sleep."

Moldofsky also found that the level of B cells, which help form antibodies, is much higher during sleep than in the waking state. He suggests that the body is rearming itself during the night to fend off invading germs the next day.

Other studies support the notion that sleep is linked to the immune system. Experiments on the clinical effects of sleep therapies have revealed that hospital patients demonstrated faster recuperation time when allowed as much sleep as they wanted. One study found that chronic fatigue and depression in older people were quickly relieved when sleep time was increased. In another, a group of women who complained of being tired, run-down, and nervous found that their symptoms either vanished or significantly lessened after a few days of longer sleep and regular naps. A second group of women, all of whom slept less than seven hours a night, were found to have five times as much tension, seven times as much fatigue, and twelve times as much nervous apprehension as their counterparts who slept at least eight hours. (In the last study, of course, it is difficult to determine whether the nervous symptoms were the *result* of sleep deprivation or the *cause* of the insomnia.)

If sleep is indeed vital to the functioning of the immune system, we now know why we are more likely to get sick if we don't get enough of it. We also know why we feel so much like sleeping when we get ill: Moldofsky found that even after being deprived of sleep for as many as 40 hours, the immune system will bounce right back to normal after a good night's sleep.

DRIFTING OFF TO REM-LAND

Perhaps because of our fascination with the content of dreams, the REM state has aroused the greatest speculation. Some say that REM provides a necessary period of stimulation for the brain, which might otherwise atrophy from the absence of stimulation over a long period of sleep. Psychoanalytic theorists, as everyone knows, have elaborate theories regarding the working out of repressed impulses, desires, and emotions, and have made an art form out of analyzing the content of dreams.

Recently, a large number of researchers have favored a more functional explanation. They believe that REM sleep is essential for consolidating memory and for assimilating traumatic experiences encountered during the day. Says Peter Hauri of the Mayo Clinic: "The function of dreaming is, in a loose sense . . . that of going over what happened during the day. We incorporate whatever has been acquired into the old stores of information, while throwing out the 'garbage,' getting rid of those things we don't really need to retain."

Many of the REM theories were generated by the finding, some time ago, that REM sleep increases after stress, worry, or new learning situations. Professor Ernest Hartmann, a leading sleep researcher and a professor of psychiatry at the Tufts School of Medicine, postulates a physiological basis for these observations. He contends that the efficiency of the synapses—microscopic areas between brain cells where impulses are transmitted from one cell to another—is restored during REM. He believes that the structural, enzymatic, and hormonal proteins produced during NREM are used for that purpose.

The speculations and the contending theories—and there are many more than the ones we mentioned—are just beginning to penetrate the mysteries of sleep. They are fascinating, and they are promising. But they are still a long way from satisfying the rigorous demands of science. Says Dr. Anthony Kales, director of a sleep research and treatment center: "When you start to ask the question, 'What is the function of sleep?' it's the same as asking, 'What is the function of wakefulness?' I don't know the function of being awake any more than I know the function of being asleep."

The interested layman might want to keep an eye on the new developments, but most insomniacs feel that the question

"Why do we sleep?" is less important than "How can I get a good night's sleep?" For most of us, it's enough to know that sleep is simply something we need, and that it is best obtained through natural means.

Somehow, the simplest things in nature are often the least amenable to the complexities of experimentation. So, until science can improve on them, we will enjoy the definitions of the poets:

> Sleep, that knits up the ravell'd sleave of care,
> The death of each day's life, sore labour's bath,
> Balm of hurt minds, great nature's second course,
> Chief nourisher in life's feast.
>
> SHAKESPEARE, *Macbeth*

THE EFFECTS OF SLEEP DEPRIVATION

In 1895, Lord Rosebery, then Prime Minister of England, resigned his office because of his chronic insomnia. In 1903 he wrote: "I cannot forget 1895. To lie, night after night, staring wide awake, hopeless of sleep, tormented in nerves, and to realize all that was going on, when I was present, so to speak, like a disembodied spirit, to watch one's own corpse, as it were, day after day, is an experience which no sane man with a conscience would repeat."

The unfortunate gentleman discovered what too many of us have learned—when you don't sleep well you suffer.

Clinical precision may be lacking as to *why* we sleep, but a good deal is known to science about what happens to those who do not get enough of it. Here are some symptoms of sleep deprivation:

- Perception deteriorates (resulting in hallucinations, if sleep loss is prolonged).
- Reaction time is damaged (interestingly, studies show that speed of reaction does not simply slow down, as we might

expect, but becomes increasingly more erratic and unpredictable, surely a greater hazard than a predictable loss of speed).

- Energy level decreases.
- Motivation diminishes.
- Vulnerability to pain increases.
- Memory becomes faulty.
- Judgment breaks down.
- Psychologically, we are apt to become negative, listless, hostile, disinterested, depressed.

Naturally, the ill effects of sleep deprivation vary from one person to another; age, physical condition, emotional well-being, and attitude all contribute to the differences. The effects will also fluctuate for each person depending on the circumstances. Sleep loss brought on by unusually stressful situations is more likely to produce severe consequences than sleep loss incurred through, say, careless overeating or travel.

To our list of scientifically proven effects of sleep loss, you can probably add your own symptoms, such as burning eyes, wobbly knees, or loss of appetite. You will doubtless recall everyday mishaps, disasters, and catastrophes linked to sleeplessness. Car accidents are a common result—studies in Oklahoma and California revealed that about 20 percent of highway accidents involved sleepy drivers; numerous other findings indicated that the sleep-deprived are less alert, less coordinated, and less able to perform simple motor tasks. Think of the loss of confidence and self-esteem, the breakdown of marriages and friendships, and regrettable misjudgments of all kinds, all traceable to unfulfilled sleep needs.

You no doubt also know the psychological difficulties to which the insomniac is heir. You can't help feeling like a freak of nature as you lie there unable to do what comes effortlessly to everyone else. "I feel injured by my insomnia," reported one sufferer, "as though I have been left out of a marvelous party that everyone else enjoys and I can only watch."

Writes another, quoted in Luce and Segal's *Insomnia:* "What hurts most about not being able to sleep is the loneliness. There you are, all alone with yourself while the rest of the world sleeps. There is nothing to distract you from your thoughts, no street noises, no TV. You're faced with yourself. There's no one who cares—no one who can care. Everybody's asleep but you."

Most of our knowledge of sleep deprivation comes from researchers who systematically aroused people during various stages of sleep. They have found that of all the stages of sleep the REM stage and to a lesser extent Stage IV are the ones we can least afford to do without. Generally speaking, a little loss of sleep here and there is compensated for easily and quickly, particularly if the loss was of Stages I, II, or III. Extensive deprivation of Stage IV, however, often results in overall lethargy, with the effects becoming more pronounced as the loss is prolonged.

Early experiments found that even a small amount of REM deprivation can lead to impairment of learning, memory, and the ability to focus. With extended loss, serious behavioral and psychological disturbances seemed to result. Subjects became confused, muddled, and found even simple tasks difficult to deal with. Eventually, it was felt, REM loss would lead to mental breakdown.

Recent evidence indicates that REM deprivation may not be quite as devastating as once believed. Many people have been found to function adequately over extended periods of time even when REM was suppressed. And in some cases depressed people seem to do better without REM sleep. Nonetheless, the overall picture is one of increasing disability the longer a person is subjected to REM deprivation.

The studies on REM loss, of course, were done under laboratory conditions, and thus the observed effects are radical. The average insomniac is hardly likely to suffer such extremes. As Dr. Charles Pollack, a prominent sleep specialist, points out, "Insomnia is not the same as being deprived of sleep in a laboratory." But the studies provide us with a useful framework for understanding what happens as a result of even mild loss of sleep. And they help explain why persons deprived of sleep will invariably have remarkably vivid dreams—and many more of them—once they finally do get some sleep.

Apparently, we need the REM stage so much that when we miss out on some we tend to spend a greater percentage of our subsequent sleep time in that stage. Called *compensatory dreaming* or *REM rebound*, this phenomenon points up the importance of the REM stage and is a significant argument against the use of sleeping pills: drugs suppress the REM stage of sleep.

As yet there is no evidence of permanent physical damage caused by prolonged sleep loss, although that possibility certainly cannot be discounted. Some scientists suspect that long-range damage may be done to the brain. However, we know so little about the brain, particularly its higher intellectual functions, that it will probably be some time before the question is settled.

AWAKE FOR 200 HOURS

In a well-publicized "wakathon" for charity, New York disc jockey Peter Tripp stayed awake for 200 hours, continuing his regular broadcasts from a glass-enclosed booth in Times Square and submitting to medical research throughout. After some time of this enforced wakefulness, Tripp began to hallucinate. A series of bizarre delusions culminated with his running naked down a hallway to escape from doctors, who, he believed, were undertakers attempting to bury him alive. He also reported a prolonged bout with depression subsequent to his vigil.

Of course, Tripp was hardly a typical insomniac. Most of us, even on our worst nights, manage to get some sleep and are hardly likely to go more than a few days without some relief. What was remarkable about Tripp's case, and others like his, was this: after a solid night's sleep, he functioned amazingly well. For the average insomniac, recovery of normal functioning is extremely quick. Even in severe cases, a period of erratic moods, plus extra time needed in compensatory sleep, are usually all the recovering individual has to contend with.

In fact, a number of experiments have shown that the body virtually demands restorative sleep when it has not gotten enough. "Given a fair chance," says one sleep expert, "the living body is naturally self-regulating and will tend to make good some temporary loss of sleep now and then by more sleep subsequently, so that on balance it gets as much natural sleep as it needs."

With respect to the effects of sleep loss, the authors have discovered a perplexing incongruity that we have labeled the Insomnia Paradox. Recalling the consequences of a bad night compels us to do all we can to ensure that we sleep well the next night. At the same time if you pay too much attention to your sleep, or to the possible consequences of losing some, you will be so anxious about not losing sleep that you will lose sleep!

Dealing with the Insomnia Paradox is a delicate matter; it requires a careful mental balancing act. Be concerned, but don't worry. Be aware of the problem, but don't belabor it. Sure, the loss of even a few hours sleep can ruin the next day. But it probably will not be as bad as you think, and you can always make up for it. Your body will insist on it.

In chapter 4 we discuss the proper attitude to adopt and give you some facts that will help you see the less gloomy side of insomnia. For now it is enough to remind you that insomnia can be easily and naturally overcome. Rest assured that, armed with the knowledge in this book, you will be able to take advantage of W. C. Fields's time-tested remedy for insomnia: "Get plenty of sleep!"

WHAT CAUSES INSOMNIA?

Mark Twain was a cantankerous insomniac. The author once found himself at a friend's home unable to sleep. The problem was not a new one to Twain, yet he convinced himself that the reason for his failure to sleep was the poor ventilation in the unfamiliar room. Unable to open the window, he tossed and turned for some time, cursing the stuffy atmosphere. Finally, in a fit of anger, he picked up his shoe and hurled it through the darkness at the window. He heard the sound of shattering glass, inhaled deeply, and then fell fast asleep. In the morning, the well-rested humorist awoke to discover that he had smashed not the window, but a glass-enclosed bookcase.

This story contains a multitude of lessons, not the least of which is that the causes we ascribe to our sleep problems may not be the real ones. It could well be that your sleep difficulties are attributable to something as simple as the ventilation in your room or to the humidity, noise, type of mattress, or what you eat and when you eat it. Such factors will be discussed in later chapters, for they definitely do affect your sleep, no matter what other elements are involved. In addition to environmental factors, situational ones also affect sleep. Everyone has experienced temporary sleep loss due to some obvious cause—jet lag, an unfamiliar bed, grief over the loss of a loved one, pressure on the job. The information in this book will help you find relief until the situation changes and normal sleep resumes.

But if you lose sleep chronically, if you often awaken unrefreshed and feel fatigued during the day, it might be a big mistake to attribute your problem only to the situation or the environment. As Mark Twain's case reveals, even the most intelligent among us find it more palatable to point the finger of blame at something outside ourselves. Safe, nonthreatening explanations are easier to live with. Unfortunately, with insomnia, they often cover up the real problems.

Failure to sleep properly is a strange and bewildering phenomenon. Unlike the failure to run fast, write well, multiply numbers easily, or bake bread, it can't be attributed to lack of skill, poor education, or insufficient talent. Everyone can sleep. Babies are terrific at it. Even dumb beasts can sleep.

If you have any doubt that it should require no great skill, talent, artifacts, or contrivances to be able to fall asleep and stay there, ask one of your deep-sleeping friends to describe how he or she does it. The person will more than likely be dumbfounded. "What do you mean, how do I go to sleep? I just do. I lie down, close my eyes, and fall asleep. That's all!"

Actually, *falling* is an apt word for it. It happens without effort or intention, just by creating a situation in which natural principles can take over—in the case of falling, gravity; in the case of falling asleep, the body's instinctive mechanisms. The person who wants to sleep well, like someone who wants to fall, must simply create a suitable situation and let go.

In its goodness, nature has made it easier to fall asleep than it is to eat. To sleep you don't need to hunt, forage, till, reap, trade, or manufacture. Indeed, the comparison indicates just how vital sleep is—we can go without food much longer than we can go without sleep.

Perhaps only breathing requires less effort than falling asleep. We don't do it; it does us. We don't go to sleep so much as sleep comes to us. We don't have to search for it—at best we coax it. Nature does all the work. It is as if our nervous systems were automatic transmissions, capable of shifting into the proper gear—waking, or the several stages of sleep— as and when they are needed.

Then why doesn't it always happen? There is no simple answer. We asked every expert we could and consulted the rest through the literature. A myriad of factors are involved, and the experts often disagree on which are the most important. In the eyes of most authorities, insomnia is not a disease, traceable to a germ or an injury or a faulty organ. Rather, it is a *sign*, an indication that the body is out of synchrony. But exactly how is hard to determine with our current state of knowledge. "We are at an early stage of defining our terms and developing a practical nosology [the classification of diseases]," says Dr. Ismet Karacan, director of the Sleep Disorders and Research Center at Baylor College of Medicine. "Proper diagnosis of a sleep disorder is difficult even with the best tools, simply because sleep is such a fragile state."

In most cases, insomnia is usually a multifaceted problem involving many aspects of our lives, interrelating and overlapping so much as to make any attempt at identifying one single cause almost arbitrary. Everything we experience affects our nervous systems and therefore our sleep. For this reason, it is difficult to guess the causes of insomnia without detailed knowledge of the individual case. Says Dr. Peter Hauri, "There might be one of a hundred things wrong with a person who can't fall asleep."

Difficulty sleeping may be rooted in an internal desynchronization, with two or more biorhythms fluctuating in periodicities that are incompatible with one another. But that is a complicated matter, about which little is known. With respect to biochemistry, the regulation of sleep may involve as many as 30 substances in a cascade of complex interactions. Precisely which chemical reactions, if any, are responsible for poor sleep is, at this time, a mystery.

Certain factors have a definite, often predictable influence on sleep, and sleep experts are trying to identify those with mathematical precision. Factors that are known to affect sleep will be discussed later in the context of the treatments that are designed to offset them. In this way, our attention will remain where it is most practical—on solutions rather than problems. Here, we will give an overview that will provide you with a perspective on the state of the art today.

The causes of insomnia fall into three categories: *physical, mental,* and *behavioral/situational.* Although sleep specialists tend, understandably, to view the problem through the narrow perspectives of their own specialties, to their credit they rarely claim to have all the answers, and they increasingly recognize the many-faceted nature of the problem. Hence, most clinics work in teams, with several disciplines represented. Unfortunately, nutrition experts or other alternative therapists are rarely found on these teams; most of the thinking tends to run along the orthodox lines of conventional physical and psychological pathologies.

With respect to the causes of insomnia, there is tremendous but good-natured disagreement among specialists. One sleep expert, a psychiatrist, estimates that 85 percent of all insomnia is due to psychiatric causes. Another psychiatrist claims that 60 percent of his patients with insomnia have major psychological problems. This is not surprising when you note that a standard psychological reference defines insomnia as "an anxiety syndrome peculiar to the neurotic personality pattern engendered by civilized society."

By contrast, a sleep expert with a different specialty— neurology—estimates that emotional problems are the cause of insomnia in only 30 percent of his patients. A physiologist feels that one third are due to psychological causes and that hidden neurological disorders cause, or aggravate, most chronic sleep troubles.

In an article in the *New England Journal of Medicine,* two psychiatrists traced sleep problems to psychological factors and advocated the use of medicine and psychotherapy as preferred treatments. In a subsequent issue, a doctor from the National Institutes of Health responded: "We cannot agree with their interpretation that psychiatric disturbances are necessarily the cause of insomnia. On the basis of their data, and that of other sleep researchers, there are at least two other interpretations, one being that the chronic sleep deprivation . . . may be the cause of the insomniac patient's psychologic disturbances. The other interpretation is that the disturbed psychologic and sleep patterns may be dual manifestations of a more fundamental disorder of physiologic activating or arousal mechanism."

In less technical terms, it is impossible to determine whether mental, physical, or other factors are the prime villains. The mind and body affect each other in a circular way.

What is interesting about the experts' opinions is that they reflect their fields of expertise even when it comes to estimating the percentage of occurrence.

TRYING TO PIN DOWN THE FACTORS

The controversy cannot be resolved yet. As the letter quoted above concluded, there is a need for continued research that would "help to elucidate the cause-and-effect relation between the psychologic and sleep disturbances as well as the long-term therapeutic value of nonpharmacologic, nontraditional psychotherapeutic treatment approaches in chronic insomnia." Specialists are, by necessity, narrow-visioned. But we can't help lamenting the loss of generalists, and we hope that the trend toward natural treatments and holistic health will soon spread to the hospitals and laboratories where they are most conspicuously absent.

Until then, the insomniac who wants to pin down the factors contributing to his or her sleep deprivation must bear in mind that each of us is a complex organism made of myriad parts, all of which affect one another.

Meanwhile, in your search for answers you might encounter the same bewilderment that befell an insomniac named Elliot Cummings. A real-estate broker whose business had recently suffered a major setback, Cummings had been losing sleep for some time. His family physician gave him a prescription for sleeping pills. Cummings did not like the side effects and gave the pills up, but he did not know where to turn next.

A friend recommended a psychoanalyst, a strict Freudian, who told Cummings that his insomnia was probably "an unconscious fear of being attacked while in a defenseless position." When Cummings suggested that the explanation was farfetched, he was offered an alternative diagnosis—he might be afraid he would walk in his sleep and attack other people.

Cummings canceled his therapy and visited another physician, who hypothesized that he was not metabolizing serotonin effectively (serotonin is a brain chemical linked with the onset of sleep). Verifying this diagnosis, however, involved a costly series of visits to a sleep clinic, which was, to Cummings, out of the question.

Cummings continued to survey the experts. A nutritionist told him he had vitamin deficiencies and poor digestion and prescribed a new diet and a plethora of supplements. Others—amateur sleuths and health faddists—suggested more causes and solutions than there are sheep to count. Bewildered, Cummings complained to a friend about his inability to come to terms with all the suggested causes. The friend offered this witty and unintentionally brilliant reply: "Sleep on it!"

Eventually, Cummings conquered his insomnia by employing a variety of treatments from vitamins to exercise. Just which ones worked is irrelevant here, since solutions vary from one person to the next. The story, however, should drive home this one point: Do not view your sleep troubles as aberrant from the rest of your 24-hour day or from your entire mental, physical, and emotional condition. This may seem obvious, but you would be surprised how many people refuse to accept it. Luce and Segal report: "Since sleep is inextricably interknit with a person's general health and way of life, it is unreasonable and illogical to expect good sleep during an inherently unhealthy life. Nonetheless, this is the expectation of most people."

Look for ways to improve your life as a whole. If your search is successful, you will find yourself sleeping more soundly. In seeking the specific roots of your sleep problem, weigh all the factors. Be vigilant and open-minded in your search for solutions. Just as you can move a table by pulling on any of its legs, you can improve your sleep by dealing with any area of your life: physical, mental, nutritional, behavioral, situational. As yet, there are no universal palliatives, no guaranteed instant cures. But, as we shall soon see, there is a veritable supermarket of effective, natural procedures to choose from without resorting to drugs.

CHAPTER 3

The Case Against Drugs

Not poppy, nor mandragora,
Nor all the drowsy syrups of the world,
Shall ever medicine thee to that sweet sleep,
Which thou owedst yesterday.
                                SHAKESPEARE, *Othello*

*S*teven Friedland, an insomniac musician, told us his experience with sleeping pills:

"I've always been one of those people whose sleep gets messed up during a crisis or an emotional upset. When I went through a particularly turbulent period, I remembered the TV commercials where insomniacs were suddenly transformed into serene Buddhas sleeping with the ease of newborn pups, and I bought some [over-the-counter] sleeping pills at my friendly pharmacy.

"On the first night, I took the recommended dosage but still could not get to sleep quickly enough to satisfy my longing. I upped the dose, figuring that since I had obtained the drug without a prescription, it could not be terribly dangerous.

"For the next three nights, I continued with the high dosage, and sure enough, I fell asleep fairly quickly. I did not feel especially good during the days, but I didn't expect to, since it was such a stressful time. On the fourth night, the pills didn't work. Thinking I must be exceptionally tense, I sweated it out.

When, a few hours later, sleep still had not come, I took some more pills, and sure enough I fell asleep. But the next day I was a mess—nauseous, dull, even more irritable than I had been.

"Alarmed that I had to exceed the recommended dosage before the pills would work, I decided to see a physician to get the *real thing*—a prescription sleeping pill. I got it with no trouble whatsoever.

" 'What's your problem?' the doctor asked.

" 'I can't sleep.'

" 'How long has this persisted?'

" 'About a week.'

" 'What have you been taking for it?'

"That was all he asked. I could see his mind linking symptom to medicine, as though he were taking a matching test in medical school.

"The drug he prescribed was a knockout. I fell asleep quickly every night for a week. I stopped passing my daytime hours worrying about whether I would fall asleep that night. True, I had indigestion, I was dull and lethargic, but I attributed all that to the crisis I was in, which was still unresolved, and to my previous lack of sleep.

"Then one night the pills didn't work. I suffered through an erratic night and a dismal day. Then it happened again. I was worried; it seemed like a relapse of my insomnia. So I took an extra pill. That did the trick. I fell asleep. The next night I didn't even bother starting out with the original dose. On the phone, the doctor okayed my decision.

"After taking the higher dose for a while, I fell prone to fits of depression, my stomach was chronically upset, I had lost a once-voracious appetite, I would incur sudden fits of the chills, and my mind was dull and disoriented. By then, the crisis that had precipitated my insomnia had pretty much been resolved. There was no reason for me to be so miserable.

"And yet, it got harder and harder to fall asleep. I was about to raise the dosage of sleeping pills again, when a friend made me recognize that I was taking too much. So I didn't take any that night. I hardly slept, and the next day I felt weak and nauseous. When I began to twitch involuntarily I went to a different doctor. Luckily, he recognized that I'd become somewhat addicted to the sleeping pills and was going through withdrawal. I had turned a mild case of situational insomnia into a real nightmare. Anyway, the doctor regulated my dosage and I got off the pills gradually. Eventually, I was myself again and I was able to sleep."

As severe as Friedland's story may seem, it is actually rather typical. Sleep medication almost invariably sets a pattern in motion: tolerance, increased dosage, tolerance, another increase in dosage, psychological dependence, physical addiction, devastating side effects, severe withdrawal symptoms—if the person even stops taking the pills. And the sad irony is that sleeping pills do not cure insomnia. Indeed, they are a perfect example of the remedy being more lethal than the malady it is designed to cure.

THE PREVALENCE OF DRUGS

During the 1970s, as many as 40 million prescriptions for sleeping pills were filled in the United States each year. Thankfully, the awareness of both insomniacs and physicians has been raised since then and the number has dropped approximately to half. Nevertheless, millions of people regularly rely on medication to fall asleep—sleeping pills are second in sales only to aspirin. The numbers increase when you consider that 75 million prescriptions for tranquilizers are filled annually, and that as much as $175 million per year is spent on over-the-counter remedies.

One doctor estimates there are enough sleeping pills produced in this country each year to put every man, woman, and child in the United States to sleep, artificially, for 200 hours. And new ones are being developed every day, even though most experts believe they are only slight variations on those already available. According to one skeptic, the drugs are being developed for the sole purpose of obtaining patents for the inventing companies.

Most doctors who have studied the matter agree that sleeping medication is dangerous and ineffective. "My feeling is that over-the-counter sleep drugs should not be sold," said Dr. Anthony Kales in an interview in the *Medical World News.* "The use and availability of these drugs is not to the advantage of the average patient."

Yet the average physician keeps on recommending them and prescribing others. Part of the problem, many experts believe, is that physicians are not given complete information on sedatives, tranquilizers, barbiturates, and other medicines due to inadequate testing, incomplete labeling, and misleading promotional literature. Research tends to limit itself to the effects of, at most, one to three days of use. Hardly any attention has been given to the long-range effects, despite the fact that over half of all prescriptions are given for periods of three months or more.

The doctor's usual source of information is the *Physician's Desk Reference,* which consists of little more than the package inserts produced by the drug manufacturers themselves. The *Reference* is really a form of advertising (in fact, drug companies spend four times as much money on promotion as they do on research). Many of the drugs are labeled "non-habit-forming," "safe," or "effective." When investigated, such claims have more often than not turned out to be exaggerated.

THE SIDE EFFECTS

Sleeping pills can cause more serious disorders than the sleeplessness they are designed to correct. According to Dr. Malcolm Lader, "All sleeping pills affect persons adversely for a minimum of eighteen hours." Here are some of the known side effects of prescription and nonprescription sleeping pills:

- impaired digestion
- circulation disorders
- blood deterioration
- respiratory problems
- blurred vision
- loss of appetite
- skin rashes
- high blood pressure
- lowered resistance to colds and infection (some pills contain ingredients known to destroy white blood corpuscles)
- dermatitis
- kidney and liver ailments
- central nervous system damage (dulling the brain)
- impaired memory
- dizziness
- irritability
- confusion
- lack of coordination
- anxiety
- depression

Obviously, there are many kinds of sleeping pills and the effects vary from one to another and from one person to another. This list was compiled without distinguishing between the various drugs and their ingredients. You should consult your physician or pharmacist for information about specific drugs.

The harmful side effects of "sleepers" are not limited to the powerful prescription drugs. Tens of millions of people make the tragic mistake of thinking that if a drug can be purchased without a prescription it must be safe. Highly advertised sleeping pills such as Nytol, Dormin, Sleep-eze, and Sominex *are* dangerous. They contain as their main sedative ingredient an antihistamine, usually methapyrilene, known by the trade name Histadyl.

One pharmacological textbook lists the following among the potential side effects of antihistamines: dizziness, incoordination, blurred vision, nervousness, anorexia, frequent urination, skin rashes, and sometimes blood changes. And although antihistamines will make a person dangerously drowsy, in the doses used in over-the-counter preparations there is little evidence that they help people fall asleep.

Scopolamine and bromides, once the most common sleeping pill ingredients and now somewhat less common, were both found toxic by a government study panel, which urged that they be banned. Of bromides, a Food and Drug Administration panel said, "The effective dose differs little from the poisonous dose." The FDA also noted that some patients who had taken too much scopolamine had been committed to psychiatric institutions with "a mistaken diagnosis of schizophrenia."

Dr. Summer M. Kalman, testifying before Congress, had this to say about bromides: "The bromides were found too dangerous for over-the-counter use because of their tendency to accumulate when used chronically and, by accumulation in the body, to pose a serious hazard to health. . . . The curious way by which bromides work—the displacement of the normal chloride ion in the body by the bromide ion so that a central nervous system depression is achieved—makes the use of these agents totally unsuitable for over-the-counter use. It is not rational for *occasional* use."

Large numbers of people with cooperative pharmacists gulp down over-the-counter tranquilizers and sleeping pills as if they were vitamins, not realizing the extent of their dependency. Frequently, the symptoms that appear—everything from irritability to hallucinations—are not linked to the drugs because their physicians don't even know their patients are using them and the patients believe they are harmless.

Each year, thousands of people die from the use of sleeping pills, both prescribed and over-the-counter. The National Institute of Mental Health estimates that one third of those deaths are not suicides. The victims die unwittingly when they carelessly have a few cocktails and soon afterward pop their pill to go to sleep. Alcohol and soporific drugs, especially barbiturates, do not mix.

Some of the deaths occur on the road, where overly sedated drivers are truly a menace. One study determined that drug users have 10 times as many accidents as do nonusers, and that 1 out of every 12 drivers is under the influence of sleeping pills or amphetamines.

Another cause of death stems from the fact that the body's tolerance for a drug varies from one moment to the next, depending on the person's physical condition, food intake, the presence of other drugs, and several other factors. The variation is so wide and so unpredictable that a small dose, sufficient to put you to sleep one day, might endanger you the next.

SLEEPING PILLS ARE ADDICTIVE

Addiction begins when the initial dosage is no longer effective in bringing on sleep. Virtually every drug tested has been shown to lose its effectiveness within two weeks (the exception, reportedly, is Dalmane, or Flurazepam, which maintains effectiveness for three to four weeks). The reason for this is that the user's body develops a tolerance for the drug, as it might for some other toxic agent. According to one expert, "We have concluded that drug dependency will develop in any medication . . . that shows a rapid development of tolerance to its sleep-inducing effects. The same principle applies to alcoholic beverages, popularly used as sleep medication."

With over-the-counter drugs the situation is particularly delicate, since they are usually not very effective in the dosage recommended on the packages. Desperate for sleep, insomniacs tend to disregard common sense and sound advice, raising the dosage arbitrarily. Because they can buy as much of the product as they want, whenever they want, they feel they are safe doing so.

Eventually, higher and higher doses are required to bring on sleep, especially when dosage is not monitored by a physician. The side effects become increasingly severe, and the users become sleeping pill junkies. Commonly, the addicted persons will take amphetamines during the day to counteract the dullness and fatigue brought on by the previous night's sleeping pills. In so doing they run the risk of having drugs dominate their entire lives, and the chances of serious and perhaps fatal consequences rise sharply.

The situation is further compounded by the users' belief that the pills are actually helping them long after their actual effectiveness has worn off. "The individual may, because he *believes* the drug is putting him to sleep, actually be able to relax enough so that he can doze off," states Dr. Peter Hauri. "But the pill itself isn't doing a thing. On the contrary, the pills are most probably going to disturb the pattern of his sleep, and his sleep is certainly going to be far more rotten because he's taken them."

Having a prescription filled and swallowing a pill or two to relieve the torment of sleeplessness hardly seems as ominous or as socially unacceptable as injecting a hypodermic needle filled with heroin. Yet, says Dr. Harris Isbell, former chief of the Public Health Service Addiction Center in Lexington, Kentucky: "Invariably, the user (of barbiturates or amphetamines) ends up a more socially destructive character than a heroin addict."

If you have been using sleeping pills for some time, and especially if you have increased your dosage, do not take these alarming facts as a signal to suddenly stop. The barbiturate habit is as difficult to break as heroin addiction. The effects of sudden withdrawal can be as dangerous and as agonizing as the celebrated "cold turkey" of the hard-core drug addict: extreme anxiety, stomach cramps, nausea, vomiting, weakness, serious weight loss, rapid breathing, fever, hallucinations, dehydration, convulsions, uncontrollable twitching, nightmares, delusions, hypertension, and, of all things, insomnia! The disruption of sleep caused by sleeping pill withdrawal is often what makes it difficult for persons to carry through with their withdrawal program. They easily convince themselves that their sleeplessness is simply a recurrence of a disease, much like getting the flu a second time in one winter. They then fall back on the pills as a way to induce sleep again.

Dr. Kales devised a way to detoxify patients without serious complications. He withdraws one clinical dose of the drug (the amount normally taken at night) once every week. The length of time of withdrawal depends, of course, on the amount of medication the person has been using and how long the person has been using it. If you use drugs regularly, Dr. Kales's method might be the best way to break the habit. The wisest step, however, is to undergo withdrawal under medical supervision. The supervision may last a long time and cost a good deal of money, but the safety factor and the benefits of being drug-independent are well worth it.

SLEEPING PILLS DISTURB SLEEP

In the 1970s, Dr. Kales, then director of the Sleep Research and Treatment Center at the Hershey Medical Center in Pennsylvania, reported a startling observation: ten insomniacs who had been using sleeping pills for some time slept as poorly as or worse than a comparable group who were receiving no medication at all. This finding gave rise to a category of illness labeled *drug-dependency insomnia*—sleeplessness actually caused by sleeping pills.

A look at how barbiturates, the most frequently used sleep-inducing chemicals, do their work will give us a better idea of why they distort normal sleep and also why they have harmful, addictive effects. This description is quoted from a pamphlet titled *Sedatives*, published by the U.S. Department of Health, Education, and Welfare:

> The principal response elicited by barbiturates is a depression of the central nervous system. They act upon the cerebral centers and interfere with the passage of impulses in the brain. They appear to affect the enzyme processes by which energy is acquired, stored in the protoplasm of the cells, and utilized. They depress brain function, and in large doses depress the brain centers responsible for maintaining the rhythm of respiration.

These drugs, then, do not induce natural sleep; they simply knock you out. The chemical processes of the brain are disrupted to the point where stuporlike unconsciousness is impossible to avoid. As Dr. Edmund Jacobson of the Laboratory for Clinical Physiology put it, sleep drugs work by "delivering a knock-out blow to the brain cells. You sleep because your nerve cells are paralyzed by what you swallow." Considering the side effects of drugs, the insomniac might be better off hitting himself over the head with a hammer.

The distinction between natural sleep and drug-induced stupor is well described in this statement by Dr. Herbert Sheldon:

> Drugs do not produce sleep. . . . In sleep the body is normally engaged in its most efficient reparative and building processes; in narcosis it is engaged in resisting and throwing off poison. This is the reason that sleep is a process of renewal and recuperation, while narcosis is an exhaustive process. The first conserves energy, the second wastes energy. Following sleep, the muscles are stronger; following narcosis the muscles are weak and tremulous. The will is weakened by narcosis; it is strengthened by sleep.

Weakness and paralysis of the nerves follow the use of narcotics; the nerves are renewed and strengthened in sleep. In sleep the heartbeat is regular; in narcosis the heartbeat is irregular, even excited. A night of sleep prepares the digestive organs for the normal performance of their functions; narcosis leaves the digestive organs weak—there is nausea, a furred tongue, loss of appetite, dyspepsia, sometimes jaundice.

Perhaps the most decisive clinical argument against drug-induced sleep is the fact that it severely interferes with the REM, or dreaming stage of sleep. Patients tend to spend a disproportionate amount of time in compensatory dreaming during their first normal sleep following a drugged sleep, the so-called REM rebound. In the case of prolonged drug-induced sleep, a veritable orgy of nightmares ensues. Although no one is quite sure why we need the REM stage so much, or what it actually accomplishes, we know enough to say that suppressing it can seriously deter the beneficial influences that arise from natural sleep.

IF YOU MUST

Steady pill taking should be avoided at all costs, if only because the pills won't work for very long. But even the staunchest antidrug crusader would not be opposed to someone taking a pill once in a great while, if one night's sleep is in question or if the person is suffering from severe pain. Dangerous as they are, pills may sometimes be used appropriately. Even Dr. Peter Hauri, an opponent of sleeping pills, does not object to their use at certain times: "If an individual is getting himself all uptight and into some sort of bind about his inability to sleep; and if this should continue for a few nights running, then he might be moving into a vicious cycle. . . . So for myself, if I start getting miserable, I'll take a sleeping pill and that will knock me out. I know, however, that the pill-induced sleep will be lousy . . . and then, the following night, I would expect the 'REM rebound.'"

If you must use medication on occasion, follow these important guidelines to minimize the danger:

- Always get a prescription from your doctor. Don't ask a friend to lend you a couple of pills. Experts say that drugs should be prescribed by a physician familiar with your medical history, taking into account the nature of your sleep disturbance and your individual physiology.

- Never try to refill a prescription without your doctor's knowledge.

- Ask your doctor what the prescribed drug's side effects are, what you can expect by way of REM rebound or other symptoms, and if there is any danger of dependency.

- If you think your doctor is too cavalier about the effects of sleeping pills, get a second opinion.

- Learn as much as you can about the drug in question. Consult Goodman and Gilman, *The Pharmacological Basis of Therapeutics,* or *Drug Information for the Consumer* from Consumer Reports Books.

- Never take pills while drinking. You might end up very sick or very dead.

- Husband and wife should not both take pills on the same night. Someone should be alert in case of an emergency.

- Do not take pills the night before a long drive or a potentially strenuous activity.

- Keep the pills away from your children. If they have trouble sleeping or are hyperactive, see your pediatrician or a child psychologist.

- Stay away from over-the-counter drugs. They are not effective and are as hazardous as prescribed medication, perhaps more so if used unsupervised.

- Of the well-tested "sleepers," some doctors lean toward Flurazepam, or Dalmane. Flurazepam apparently does not reduce REM sleep as many other drugs do, but it does reduce Stage III and IV sleep.

The most sensible approach to sleeping pills is to leave them on your pharmacist's shelf. In the following chapters you will find a comprehensive potpourri of safe, nonpharmaceutical procedures for helping you restore natural sleep. With a little patience and some trial and error, you are likely to find a combination that will work for you.

CHAPTER 4

Your Body and Your Sleep: The Medical Factor

*I*f you have chronic sleep problems, the first thing you should do is see a physician to determine whether or not medical factors are in any way responsible. Insomnia has been linked clinically with both serious pathologies and minor disorders, as well as the use of drugs. This chapter will make you aware of possible medical causes of insomnia, which you might not otherwise consider. The methods discussed throughout the remainder of the book will probably help you with your problem regardless of its cause, but be sure to see your doctor or a sleep specialist if you suspect that medical factors are interfering with your sleep.

One possible cause of insomnia is a respiratory disorder. Asthma sufferers, for example, and often awakened by attacks in the night, usually in the earlier stages of sleep. Asthmatics should not take sleeping pills under any circumstances, as they depress the respiratory control centers in the brain, compounding breathing difficulties. Moderate (not vigorous) afternoon exercise has been recommended in such cases because it seems to increase the percentage of time spent in Stages III and IV of sleep. However, this is inconclusive, and is certainly not to be taken as a treatment for the asthma itself.

Coronary patients are often stricken with attacks of angina pectoris (chest pains) that awaken them during the night. According to one study, about 80 percent of these nighttime attacks occur during REM sleep. Medication is commonly used to treat angina, since it can enlarge the blood vessels, but doctors advise against the use of any drugs that suppress REM sleep. That, of course, includes sleeping pills. The REM rebound that occurs subsequent to REM loss may increase the risk of angina attacks in these patients.

Other medical problems known to contribute to sleep difficulties include ulcers, migraine and cluster headaches, hyperthyroidism, hypothyroidism, arthritis, diabetes, kidney disease, epilepsy, and Parkinson's disease. Naturally, any serious illness is going to affect sleep in some way. The ones mentioned here are known to interfere with sleep directly, and often without the insomniac's realizing it. Your attending physician should be made aware of your sleep problem.

PHYSIOLOGICAL CONDITIONS THAT CAN DISRUPT SLEEP

Several forms of pathology that occur during sleep are known to contribute to insomnia. These can usually be diagnosed only in a sleep laboratory. You may go to your regular doctor with complaints of interrupted sleep or constant fatigue but, unless he is familiar with the latest sleep research, he will rarely suspect one of these disorders.

Sleep apnea is a syndrome in which abnormal respiratory function during sleep prevents adequate breathing. Found in approximately 5 percent of the patients who visit sleep clinics, apnea often goes undetected for years. In this affliction, the body's automatic control of breathing breaks down as it shifts from waking to sleep. Sometimes the breathing will cease for as long as a minute. The person awakens with a start and gasps for air with a loud snore.

This can be repeated as many as 400 to 500 times a night, but the interruptions are usually so brief that the victims are totally unaware of them. All they know is that they do not sleep well, they are groggy and drowsy all day, and their families complain about their loud snoring.

Researchers are not in agreement about whether apnea is a cause of insomnia. The illness may be entirely unrelated to "difficulty initiating or maintaining sleep." In any event, the disorder is more common than anyone believed a few years ago. If our description of apnea sounds familiar, you are well-advised to see a knowledgeable doctor, who will either observe your sleep in his office or refer you to a sleep clinic where all-night monitoring can determine whether or not you have the disorder. If you are over 40 and if you have a tendency toward obesity, the chances are greater that you may have it.

In some cases apnea can be treated with medication. However, the most successful cure is rather drastic—a type of tracheotomy, a surgical incision in the windpipe that permits unobstructed breathing during sleep and is covered during the day.

Nocturnal myoclonus is another insomnia-causing sleep pathology. One study connected myoclonus to 10 to 20 percent of chronic insomnia cases. In this disorder the legs jerk abruptly every 25 to 40 seconds in a periodic manner. Attacks may last for minutes or for hours. The jerking will arouse the sleeper as many as 400 times a night, but the person may not be aware of the cause.

If your spouse complains of being kicked in the night, if you often have discomfort in your lower leg muscles, or have "restless leg syndrome" (an inability to keep your legs still while lying awake), you should see your physician or a sleep specialist for advice.

Doctors are still searching for a cure for myoclonus. Some drugs have shown promise, but not to the degree hoped for. Nonetheless, it is important to determine whether or not you have this disorder, and whether it is serious enough to warrant treatment.

Circadian rhythm disturbance is a category of sleep disorder that causes apparent insomnia. Some people seem to suffer from something roughly analogous to permanent jet lag. Their biological rhythms are chronically out of phase with their social environments, or their cycles are longer than the normal 24 hours. They might, for example, have cycles that last 25 to 27 hours. After a week, what is still 8 o'clock in the evening to everyone else can be 2 o'clock in the morning to them.

These people sleep normally, but at the "wrong times," in relation to the 24-hour day that ordinary social and business conventions require. If they are aware of the nature of the difficulty (most of them are not, for it simply seems to them that frequently they can't get to sleep), and if their professional schedule and family life enable them to sleep and wake at unconventional times, then the problem can be solved easily.

But that is rare. Sleep researchers, newly aware of this problem, are investigating ways to recondition those out-of-sync rhythms. One promising method consists of confining the patient to an environment in which there are no outer stimuli—no windows, clocks, schedules, or other infringements. Once the person's individual pattern is recognized, the doctors can then reprogram his or her sleep/wake rhythms by systematically adjusting the time the patient goes to sleep.

MEDICATIONS AS MYSTERIOUS INSOMNIA INDUCERS

The use of drugs other than sleeping pills is another sleep-robber that often goes undetected and requires medical attention in most cases. Here are three revealing cases.

An insomniac artist named Ed Crane was wise enough to avoid sleeping pills because he had heard about their side effects. Unfortunately, he was not as discriminating about the amphetamines he was taking to stimulate his tired body into action during the day, nor about the antidepressant drugs he was taking to overcome "the blahs." Like most drug users, he did not realize that the pills he thought would counteract the effects of sleep loss were actually interfering with his sleep. It took a last-resort visit to a doctor who specialized in sleeping disorders to enlighten him.

Then there was the woman we interviewed who suffered insomnia, mysteriously enough, only in late summer and early fall. She was bewildered by this predictable pattern. Finally she discovered the reason behind it. A sufferer of severe allergies, she had been in the habit of taking large doses of antihistamines during the hay fever season—late summer and early fall. One year, fed up with the drowsiness the pills induced, she stopped using them. Her experiment did nothing for her hay fever symptoms, but a remarkable thing happened: she began to sleep better.

Confused, she consulted a doctor. Fortunately, the doctor had done his homework. He knew that antihistamines, like tranquilizers and amphetamines, can lead to the same difficulties we described in the chapter on sleeping pills.

Karen Elder is a young woman who began to have sleep problems about the time she was married. Disturbed by the coincidence, she wondered if sharing a bed with her husband or perhaps some deep, unconscious neurosis stirred up by marriage might be responsible. She became so despondent about the latter possibility that she went to a psychologist.

Still, she did not sleep as well as she once did. Then one day she read a report on the alleged dangers of birth-control pills, which she had been taking since her marriage. Concerned, she switched to another contraceptive method. Soon she began sleeping well again. It seems that female sex hormones influence the pituitary gland and the sleep center in the brain. The Pill can alter hormonal balance enough to affect sleep— sometimes causing the woman to sleep more, sometimes less.

Drugs used in connection with medical problems are usually prescribed by a physician. For that reason, and because these compounds are so powerful, patients who suspect that such drugs are interfering with their sleep should consult with their doctors before abandoning the medication outright. If your physician is not sympathetic to your desire to cut down or eliminate a drug, or if he doesn't agree with your suggestion that a medication might be interfering with your sleep, consider getting a second opinion.

In some cases a trade-off will be necessary. If the drug is, in fact, interfering with your sleep but is needed for medical purposes, you and your doctor will have to decide whether the loss of sleep is good enough reason to give it up. In some cases the drug can be discontinued in favor of an alternative that does not disturb sleep.

THE ANTI-SLEEP EFFECT OF SMOKING AND DRINKING

According to an article in the *Medical Tribune*, heavy smokers have a harder time falling asleep and spend less time in the important Stage IV and REM states than do nonsmokers. The article further stated that when they gave up the habit, the former smokers were able to fall asleep faster, sleep longer with fewer interruptions and, after a period of compensation, have the normal amount of REM sleep.

Nicotine is a stimulant. If you are a heavy smoker, and particularly if you wake up craving a smoke, it is possible that cigarettes contribute to your problem. Needless to say, you ought to stop smoking to prevent disorders that are far more dangerous than some lost sleep. At the very least, you will want to cut down in the hours before bedtime.

How to stop, or at least cut down? As anyone who has tried knows, it isn't easy. Your doctor might be a good first stop, although many physicians are at a loss to offer anything more than encouragement. Behavioral psychologists, hypno-therapists, acupuncturists—these and other therapists have claimed success in helping people stop smoking. There are many organizations, as well as books and tapes (for example, "Larry Hagman's Stop Smoking For Life" video) that promise relatively painless ways to kick the habit. SmokEnders has had more than 30,000 graduates and claims that only 6 of every 100 ever smoked again. (For more information write SmokEnders' World, Phillipsburg, NJ 08865.)

As for alcohol, although mild social drinking appears to be relatively harmless and a wine nightcap might even be a safe soporific, large amounts of booze can be devastating to sleep. Once alcohol is metabolized, the body goes into a state of withdrawal, which can arouse the sleeper. In addition, alcohol tends to increase the production of urine, which can awaken the sleeper with the need to dash to the bathroom.

According to a publication from the Sleep/Wake Disorders Unit at New York's Montefiore Hospital, "The sleep of alco-holics is characterized by many nighttime awakenings, low total sleep time, lower than normal amounts of Stage III or IV of Non-REM and of REM sleep, and a higher frequency of changes between states and stages of sleep." In other words, alcohol makes sleep erratic. The irony is that many heavy drinkers originally took to the bottle in order to help a sleep problem. Then they gradually stepped up their intake to combat the body's growing tolerance and eventually became habituated. Some doctors postulate that alcoholism may permanently disturb the sleep mechanism.

As is the case with other drugs, sudden withdrawal from alcohol can be hazardous. Your doctor or the local chapter of Alcoholics Anonymous should be consulted if you are addicted to alcohol and want to stop drinking. Heavy drinkers who wish to cut down but not abstain entirely, or to whom an occasional drink seems to be a professional or social necessity, may find help without being labeled alcoholics from an organization called Drinkwatchers, headquartered in Burlingame, California.

These medical factors are probably responsible for only a fraction of sleep difficulties; in the great majority of cases, it is impossible to pinpoint one specific physiological cause. In their search for universal factors that might be present in all cases of insomnia, researchers have been probing the biochemical parameters of sleep. So far, the most significant finding has been the isolation of the brain chemical *serotonin*, which is involved in the onset of sleep. Scientists speculate that insomniacs may have difficulty converting serotonin from its amino acid precursor, *l-tryptophan*. (See chapter 5 for more on l-tryptophan.) Degeneration of brain cells in particular regions has also been mentioned as a possible universal factor, but so far nothing conclusive has been discovered.

One general factor that probably causes or contributes to the nervous system's inability to shift properly into and out of sleep is stress. What that is, and how to deal with it, is covered in chapter 5.

OBTAINING MEDICAL HELP

Although the overwhelming majority of physicians, unaware of the latest research on sleep, still treat insomnia by dispensing sleeping pills, a growing number are inclined toward less harmful alternatives. You might want to seek a physician with such an orientation.

An even better alternative might be to seek out a sleep specialist, particularly if you suffer from extreme daytime sleepiness or if your insomnia is accompanied by difficulty breathing, violent leg movements, or a level of snoring that disturbs your spouse. Sleep disorders as a clinical specialty grew tremendously in the 1980s as research on sleep expanded and new diagnostic procedures were introduced. If your case warrants specialized attention, you might be referred to a sleep disorders center. In 1978, when the first edition of this book was published, there were 6 accredited sleep disorders centers in the United States. There are now more than 100, with hundreds more in various stages of development.

You can be confident that the staff and consultants at a sleep disorders center are abreast of the latest research. They are also uniquely equipped to diagnose unusual disturbances such as sleep apnea and nocturnal myoclonus, and to treat special cases that require sophisticated equipment. If you enroll at a sleep clinic, you will typically be asked to keep a log of your sleep patterns before your first visit. You will then be interviewed by a sleep specialist and asked to fill out extensive questionnaires regarding your medical history and other pertinent information. After a complete physical examination, you might be advised to spend a night or two at the center, where state-of-the-art instruments will analyze your sleep. The staff will then evaluate all the data and recommend a program of treatment.

One of the authors of this book enrolled as a patient at the Sleep/Wake Disorders Center at Montefiore Medical Center in New York. I found the experience not only painless but enlightening. The physicians and staff were uniformly supportive and pleasant, the facility sparkling clean, the attention comprehensive. Although the mystery of my insomnia was not clarified unequivocally, there was something reassuring about seeing the chart of my brain waves and other physiological functions during my sleep, and in the opportunity to discuss my condition at length with experts. The solution to my insomnia eventually lay in diet and exercise, but I walked away from the clinic with excellent advice and the comforting knowledge that my condition was not nearly as serious as I'd imagined it was.

Treatment at a sleep disorders center is expensive, but so is taking sleeping pills, the loss of productivity due to poor sleep, and the possibility of minor mishaps and major accidents when you walk and drive in a stupor. According to Dr. Elliot Weitzman, the former director of the Montefiore Center, "We find that it's much less than the patient paid before being taken care of, not only for pills, but wrong diagnoses, or inadequate therapy—I mean thousands of dollars." If your problem is severe enough, your insurance company might cover the cost of the diagnosis and treatment.

Bear in mind that sleep clinics are not infallible; their success rate is hardly perfect. Says Dr. Charles Pollack, a former codirector of the Montefiore Center: "The patients' expectations are usually too high. They expect a magic cure. Often they don't have the willingness to do anything from their side." He adds, however, that physicians sometimes *raise* the patients' expectations because the patients don't believe they can be helped.

For a current listing of accredited sleep disorders facilities, contact The American Sleep Disorders Association, 604 2nd St. SW, Rochester, MN 55902; (507) 287-6006.

ALTERNATIVE MEDICAL SOURCES

In recent years, alarmed by what is perceived as an overreliance on drugs and insufficient emphasis on prevention, growing numbers of people have been seeking alternative healing procedures not just for insomnia but for many ailments. Of the drugless systems of medicine that are gaining favor, several have received good reports from people with sleep problems. Here are brief descriptions of four:

Chiropractic

The days when most people thought of chiropractors as "bone doctors" or "back crackers" seem to be over. Chiropractors, who consider themselves nerve specialists and holistic practitioners, are rigorously trained doctors who typically employ a wide range of natural treatments—nutrition, hydrotherapy, exercise, and so forth—but whose special training is in adjusting the vertebrae of the spinal column.

According to chiropractic theory, misalignment of the vertebrae can interfere with the activity of the nervous system, since it is from the spinal column that nerves branch out to the brain and to all the organs and glands of the body. Chiropractors believe that the nervous system regulates the body's natural healing powers. By removing impediments to its proper functioning, they feel we can enable the body to cure, or at least hasten recovery from, disease.

Several insomniacs we interviewed claimed that occasional chiropractic adjustments have helped their sleep. They reported feeling less tense for some period after an adjustment. Chiropractors can also help with posture problems that might interfere with sleep, and they are often excellent sources of advice on nutrition and referrals to other natural practitioners. If you think a dysfunction of nerves, blood flow, or other organic process is causing your insomnia, it is possible that chiropractic treatments will help clear the way to a good night's sleep.

A recommendation by a physician is the best way to find a good chiropractor. Failing that, health-conscious acquaintances are a good source. In addition, most states have chiropractic associations and licensing boards that can supply you with the names of practitioners in your location. For additional information, contact the American Chiropractic Association, 2200 Grand Ave., Des Moines, IA 50312; or the International Chiropractic Association, 741 Brady St., Davenport, IA 52808.

Homeopathy

Homeopathy is based on the "law of similars," which may be summarized as "like is cured by like." Homeopathic procedures are much the same, in theory, as the use of vaccines—they stimulate symptoms so the body can strengthen its capacity to purge itself of illness. After conducting a detailed interview to discern the full range of the patient's symptoms, the homeopathic practitioner prescribes a remedy that would produce a similar set of symptoms in a well person. These remedies, derived from plant, animal, and mineral sources, contain infinitesimal quantities of minerals found in the body, such as sodium, potassium, iron, calcium, magnesium, phosphorus, sulfur, and iodine. The proper compound in the correct dosage will relieve the symptoms—sometimes quickly, sometimes gradually—with no side effects.

Like chiropractic, homeopathy has its detractors in the medical community. However, it remains in good repute in European countries and is now enjoying a resurgence in the United States, where it was once a thriving specialty. A growing number of qualified homeopathic practitioners is setting up shop, and many conventionally trained physicians dispense homeopathic remedies in addition to standard medicines. Although little scientific research has been done on its procedures, that which has been done has been encouraging. Furthermore, homeopathy appears to be harmless—when the treatments don't work, they just don't work, but they are nontoxic, will produce no known side effects, and are not habit-forming.

A widely used homeopathic textbook lists several remedies for insomnia, including: *coffea cruda,* for someone whose sleep is disturbed by mental activity and nervous excitability; *cypripedium*, particularly for young children; *daphne indica*, for someone with a severe inability to sleep, along with nightmares, chills, and clamminess; *ignatia*, for insomnia caused by grief and cares and characterized by jerking limbs; *passiflora incarnata*, for restless and wakeful sleep caused by worry and overwork; *aquilegia*, for insomnia with nervous trembling and sensitivity to light and noise. One homeopathic physician's favorite remedy for insomnia is a dose of "homeopathic coffee" an hour or two before bedtime, then another dose just before bed. Finally, *calms forte*, a common homeopathic compound, is often recommended for temporary relief of anxiety and sleeplessness.

Homeopathic remedies, which are taken orally, can be obtained over the counter in certain pharmacies; some are available at health-food stores. But the best way to proceed is to have a personal consultation with a qualified homeopathic practitioner, who will prescribe a regimen according to an overall assessment of your condition. You can obtain a list of trained homeopaths from the National Center of Homeopathy, 1500 Massachusetts Ave. NW, Ste. 41, Washington, DC 20005; (202) 223-6182. Or, the International Foundation for Homeopathy, 2366 Eastlake Ave. East, Seattle, WA 98102; (206) 324-8230.

Ayurvedic Medicine

The term *ayurveda* in Sanskrit means "the science of life." The system of medicine that bears this name is probably the oldest in the world, dating to 500 B.C. according to some sources and as far back as 3000 B.C. according to others. Ayurveda is still used widely throughout India, and in fact is enjoying a resurgence not only in Asia but in the United States and Europe.

Ayurveda is principally oriented toward prevention, its underlying aim being to promote a state of perfect physiological balance. Taking into account mental and spiritual factors as well as physical signs and symptoms, ayurveda uses a wide variety of natural procedures and herbal-based natural remedies. The emphasis is on treating the individual as a whole as opposed to only his or her specific symptoms. Different people reporting similar cases of insomnia might, subsequent to an ayurvedic examination, be given different treatment programs.

Fundamental to the ayurvedic system is the concept of *doshas*, three basic metabolic principles that are said to govern our physiology. The three *doshas* are: *vata*, which is responsible for all movement in the body; *pitta*, which produces energy and heat, and governs digestion; and *kapha*, which provides the body's substance and solidity. The goal of ayurveda is to create balance among these three forces. The *doshas* are further used to identify each person's body type. Ayurvedic physicians use a number of diagnostic procedures and a medical history to determine the patient's body type and outline an appropriate treatment program.

The regimen might entail any of a variety of procedures, including yogic exercises, meditation, purification practices, and dietary recommendations. In addition, specific sleep-promoting procedures might be recommended: drinking certain herbal teas before bed, aroma therapies using plant-based scents, massage, and such esoteric pre-bed items as massaging the feet with *ghee* (clarified butter) and applying to the forehead a paste made of sandalwood powder, nutmeg, and camphor in warm water.

Some major population centers have trained ayurvedic practitioners in their vicinities. Your best course is to ask at a health-food store or holistic health clinic, or consult the listings in publications that feature alternative medicine. The Transcendental Meditation organization has several ayurvedic centers in the United States, staffed by Western-trained medical doctors who have also had special training in ayurveda. They will gear a treatment program to your individual condition. Their universal recommendations for sleep include several practices that are consistent with advice reported elsewhere in this book. In addition, they suggest the following nonmedicinal sleep aids if one is needed: saffron heated in milk; a large pinch of nutmeg stirred into warm milk; a quarter- to a half-teaspoon of poppy seed stirred into a cup of warm water.

For the address of a Maharishi Ayurveda Center near you, write P.O. Box 282, Fairfield, IA 52556; (515) 472-5866.

Chinese Medicine: Acupuncture and Herbs

In recent years, the practice of acupuncture has attracted a good deal of attention as a drugless method of performing anesthesia and treating pain. However, Chinese medicine is a lot more than acupuncture, and its repertoire of procedures has been gaining repute in the West. A number of Americans have earned doctorates in Oriental Medicine from accredited colleges, and an even larger number have become licensed acupuncturists.

Chinese medicine is rooted in the ancient philosophical system of Taoism. In the ancients' view, nature as a whole is characterized by unity, yet all objects and processes are in constant and rhythmic flux, shifting from one polarity to the other in an effort to achieve harmony. The two poles are Yin (passive, yielding, and nurturing, feminine) and Yang (dynamism, rationality, and masculinity). One ancient saying goes: "The Yin conserves and the Yang radiates."

With respect to health, Yin is associated with substance—the material properties of the body—whereas Yang is the energy that allows the body to function. According to Santa Monica, California acupuncturist Elizabeth Sandler, trouble sleeping means not enough Yin or too much Yang. Yin is associated with the night, when Yang is drawn into the Yin of the body, allowing us to rest. Says Sandler: "Insomnia is a symptom of some physiological imbalance. The goal of Chinese medicine is to restore that balance."

If you see a practitioner of Chinese medicine for your insomnia, he or she will probably take a complete medical history and inquire about various aspects of your life that may be affecting your sleep. In addition, the practitioner is likely to perform either a pulse diagnosis or a tongue diagnosis, or both. These are time-honored procedures said to reveal a great deal about inner conditions. Based on the overall picture, the practitioner will prescribe an individual regimen of acupuncture and herbs.

Acupuncture is the now-familiar practice of inserting small needles in specific points, or energy vortexes, along *meridians*, or energy pathways. The practice, which is virtually painless, redirects the flow of energy and blood, enabling the body's natural healing tendencies to restore balance. In addition to acupuncture, the practitioner will probably prescribe herbal remedies from the elaborate pharmacopoeia in the Chinese tradition.

Finding a qualified acupuncturist may be as simple as flipping through the Yellow Pages. If that doesn't work, find out if your state has licensing procedures for acupuncturists and contact the licensing board for a referral. Or, contact the National Commission for the Certification of Acupuncturists, 1424 16th St. NW, Ste. 501, Washington, DC 20036; (202) 232-1404. They will provide a list of licensed practitioners in your area.

In lieu of a licensed practitioner, you might help yourself the Chinese way with self-administered *acupressure*, which substitutes manual manipulation for needles. In chapter 9 we include simple instructions for using acupressure in bed when you have trouble sleeping.

You can also help yourself to Chinese herbal remedies. We spoke to Ron Teeguarden, a well-known expert and practicing herbologist. Teeguarden, author of the book *Chinese Tonic Herbs*, says that the proper herbs will help to regulate the body's natural sleep/wake rhythms. He recommends either of two herbal combinations to be taken morning and night in capsule form. These are not sedatives, but tonic herbs, used for restorative purposes. They will not only reduce the nervous nighttime energy that disturbs sleep, he says, but will enhance energy and vitality during the day. These classic formulas are prepared and freeze-dried in Taiwan by either Jen-On Enterprises or Sun-Ten Pharmaceuticals.

For people with difficulty falling asleep, the *ginseng and longan* combination is recommended; for those who can't stay asleep, the *ginseng and zizyphus* combination. Both formulas are said to be safe and non-habit-forming, and both are available with *codonopsis* instead of ginseng if the latter proves too energizing (codonopsis is often recommended over ginseng for women). The formulas are not cheap, but once they fulfill their stated promise of reestablishing the body's natural biorhythms their use can be discontinued.

For temporary relief from insomnia, more sedative herbs can be used. One combination, Schizandra Dreams, contains kava kava, amber, and other sleep-promoting herbs. Alternatively, herbs can be purchased in bulk and brewed as tea. Teeguarden recommends zizyphus and polygala, either separately or together. Make a gallon or two, boil the herbs for about an hour, strain, and refrigerate. Then simply heat a cup before bed as needed.

For bulk herbs, the best place to shop is the nearest China-town. The combination formulas can be obtained from an herbalist or a professional acupuncturist. They can also be ordered through the mail. For a catalog, write: The Tea Garden Herbal Emporium, 1344 W. Washington Blvd., Venice, CA 90291.

A few caveats regarding alternative systems of medicine:

- Just as there are cynics who will denigrate these systems, accuse them of quackery, and try to steer you away, there are zealots, fanatics, and outright charlatans who will lay claim to the most outrageous feats on behalf of their favorite practitioner. Be wary of extremists on both ends. The truth usually lies somewhere in the middle.

- Make sure the practitioner you go to has been properly trained and licensed.

- Be aware that your health insurance might not cover alternative practices, and if it does the coverage might be limited. Many practitioners work with or under the auspices of M.D.s; this usually renders the billing more acceptable to insurance companies.

CHAPTER 5

Stress and Sleep: How to Relieve Stress and Tension

*T*he character of modern life—with its pressures, changes, pollutants, noise, overstimulation, and manifold nuisances—can wreak havoc on the endocrine and nervous systems, throwing the body's natural rhythms out of balance. The result can be a disruption of your natural sleep rhythms.

Since its importance was first recognized and defined by the late Dr. Hans Selye in the 1960s, *stress* has been studied by dozens of researchers. We know quite precisely how it affects our bodies, our minds, and, by extension, our sleep. The General Adaption Syndrome, first described by Dr. Selye, works in this way: When a stressful situation occurs—an attack by a mugger, a reprimand from your boss, a traffic jam, or even something pleasant but overwhelming, such as winning a lottery or walking into a room and having a hidden crowd yell "surprise!"—the adrenal and pituitary glands begin to secrete hormones that both protect the body from injury and muster up strength from stored sugars and fats. Energy is mobilized, respiration and blood pressure rise, muscles tense, pupils dilate. These and other automatic responses are instilled in us by nature to prepare the threatened body for either fight or flight.

Our ancestors had everyday stressors that required violent reactions—attacks by wild beasts, for example—but most contemporary stressors require neither fleeing nor fighting. Our highly mobilized bodies do not *use* the powerful resources that are summoned. And if we stifle the emergency response too often, the result can be more-or-less permanent damage to tissues and organs, and an overall weakening of the endocrine and nervous systems. Hence, stress is literally "the wear and tear caused by life."

In extreme cases, heart disease, hypertension, or any of a number of serious psychosomatic illnesses can result from stress directly. For most of us, however, general tension is the result. It is as though the body were in a state of perpetual mobilization.

Undoubtedly, stress-induced imbalances affect the ability to sleep properly. As far back as 1976, *The Journal of Human Stress* reported clinical studies in which stress factors were found to disturb sleep. One showed a decrease in Stage IV sleep; another showed measurable REM disturbance after the subjects were exposed to stressful situations. A more recent study found that during the year their sleep problems began, chronic insomniacs experienced a greater number of stressful life events compared with previous or subsequent years. They also tended to have less satisfying relationships, lower self-concepts, and more discontent than non-insomniacs. This should not be surprising. Stress creates an aroused, hypermetabolic state; sleep is an *un*aroused, *hypo*metabolic state.

In the last decade, the search for ways to combat stress has become increasingly prolific; relaxation techniques, exercise, high-tech gadgetry, and unorthodox medical practices have all emerged. In this chapter we will discuss a variety of procedures that are advocated as ways to alleviate the effects of stress. We selected those that have acquired good reputations and have demonstrated a beneficial influence on sleep.

Where possible we provide step-by-step instructions that you can follow on your own, immediately. In cases where the services of trained experts are required, we provide enough information for you to understand the subject and to locate the appropriate assistance.

RELAXATION THERAPY

Tension is insomnia's dance partner, both leading and following sleeplessness. It can keep you awake at night, and then, as a result of the loss of sleep, appear the next day in the form of nervousness, worry, anxiety, and fear. Therefore, eliminating tension from both the external muscles and the visceral muscles—the muscles of the internal organs—is an important step toward acquiring sound sleep.

Doctors have concluded that most people have some neuromuscular tension, detectable by instruments even when they think they are completely relaxed. You have probably noticed that even when lying perfectly still in bed your muscles maintain a certain degree of rigidity. Prior to sleep, your muscles should be limp, not rigid.

A great number of techniques have been developed for relaxing those tense muscles. Most involve efforts of the mind, and many of those seem overly strenuous. Without proper supervision, some instructions given by well-meaning writers can result in persons straining their minds in an attempt to achieve relaxation. Stay away from anything that might lead to strain, for that, obviously, will have the opposite effect from the one intended—it will make you tense.

Of the techniques that seem safe and potentially effective, one of the most popular is Progressive Relaxation, developed in the 1940s by Dr. Edmund Jacobson of the Laboratory for Clinical Physiology. Progressive Relaxation involves learning to recognize the signs of muscular contraction and cultivating the ability to eliminate increasingly deeper levels of tension.

In *How to Sleep Well*, Dr. Samuel Gutwirth, a student of Dr. Jacobson's, writes: "Insomnia is always accompanied by a sense of residual tension and can always be surmounted when one is successful in discontinuing contraction of the muscles even in this minute degree. Abolishing residual tension is, then, the essential feature in learning to relax scientifically."

Here are the basic instructions for Progressive Relaxation:

Once a day, set aside practice periods of 45 minutes to an hour, just before or just after a meal. Arrange not to be disturbed. Loosen your clothing. Lie down on a wide bed or couch in a quiet room (it need not be dark) with your arms at your side, palms down, several inches from your body. Do not fold your hands or cross your legs. Close your eyes gently and easily—do not try to shut them tightly.

Now relax by letting your weight sink into the bed. Do not *try* to relax, do not try talking to yourself in order to facilitate settling down. Dr. Gutwirth makes a point of distinguishing this method from autosuggestion. After about 10 minutes, slowly stiffen the muscles in both arms without moving your arms and without clenching your fists. The stiffening should be done slowly, without putting undue stress on the muscles. Hold at a slight degree of stiffness for about 10 seconds. Now stiffen a little more and hold for another 10 seconds. Again stiffen and hold, this time for about 30 seconds.

Carefully observe how your arms feel. You should notice a dull, taut sensation. This is indicative of contracted muscles and active nerves. Becoming aware of this sensation—the signs of muscular tension—is the first step in relaxation therapy.

Now allow your arms to relax slowly, a little at a time. Notice how the taut sensation begins to diminish in intensity. Enjoy this relaxed state for 5 minutes.

Repeat the entire procedure—stiffening and holding

in progressive stages, becoming aware of the sensations, and then slowly relaxing.

Repeat a third time.

After the third repetition, continue to let your arms relax. Relax them further and further, past the point where they felt relaxed initially.

Relaxation therapy is the opposite of an exercise or an activity during which the muscles are contracted. It is a procedure of doing less and less. The key is to *let* yourself relax, not to *make* yourself relax.

Once you have mastered the procedures above, do the same with other muscle groups—the legs, chest, abdomen, and facial muscles. Always tense them and relax them in the same systematic manner that you followed with your arms. After a while you will be able to achieve a deep state of muscular relaxation. Soon you'll also be able to discontinue the period of tensing that precedes the relaxation. However, it's best to do it at first in order to become acquainted with the contrasting sensations of tension and relaxation. Eventually, though, you should be able to lie down and completely relax every muscle group without effort.

According to Dr. Jacobson, the muscles of the eyes and face are particularly important for those who have sleep difficulties. They are, customarily, among the last muscles groups to become relaxed. "When any person lies without sleeping," says Dr. Jacobson, "it is because he is using his eyes and his speech to imagine or to recall, to think, to solve problems or to engage in other forms of mental activity. I have found that if eyes and speech organs are really relaxed (as measured electronically) for even as short a time as 30 seconds, the person is asleep at the end of this time."

Here are two techniques for relaxing the eye and face muscles:

Lie down as before and, with eyelids closed, wrinkle your forehead by pulling up your eyebrows. Hold this position for about a minute, familiarizing yourself with the feeling of tension in the forehead muscles. Then let the forehead relax gradually. Hold the muscles in this relaxed state for about 5 minutes. Now close your eyelids very tightly. Hold in that position for about 30 seconds, noting the tension in the eyelids. Then let your eyelids go. Relax for a few minutes. Do this repeatedly until you feel all the residual tension is gone. As in the other procedures, the initial period of tensing up can eventually be eliminated.

Another technique for relaxing the eyes can be done at bedtime. Close your eyelids tightly and, without moving your head, look up. Hold this position for about 30 seconds, observing the tension in your eye muscles and eyeballs. Now relax your eyes completely, letting them go limp in their sockets. Lie in this relaxed state for about 5 minutes. Repeat the entire process. Next, close your eyes tightly, but this time look *down*. Again, do not move your head. Follow the usual procedure for noticing the sensations and then relaxing. Do the same by looking to the right and to the left, always with eyes tightly closed and the head stationary.

Dr. Gutwirth reported great success with the methods described above. He claimed that after a few weeks of practice, insomniacs found it easy to let go and relax when they went to bed.

Dr. Peter Hauri of the Mayo Clinic reported good results with some patients using Progressive Relaxation. He saw essentially two benefits in the method. As the first benefit, it "actually does help a person to relax tense muscles. It is absolutely essential that a chronically tense person learn to relax. The longer some people stay in bed, the more tense they get. PR helps them eliminate that tension."

The second virtue is indirect, according to Dr. Hauri: "Actually, the majority of insomniacs are not chronically tense. The way in which PR helps these people is to keep their minds occupied with something else so that the body will naturally relax. The PR exercises will distract them enough so that they will not *try* to sleep, which is the worst thing an insomniac can do."

Dr. Hauri adds, however, that PR is "not always useful for my insomniac patients." He uses biofeedback, meditation, and "whatever technique the patient has least resistance to." In some cases, he said, his Progressive Relaxation people "try so hard to relax with the PR that they get exhausted"—the kind of exhaustion that does not lead to sleep.

Overall, Progressive Relaxation is a highly regarded technique for simple muscle relaxation. When you try it, remember to let go—don't strain trying to relax.

MEDITATION

Once regarded as mystical and obscure or as a counterculture fad, meditation has become better understood in recent years and is now accepted as a legitimate method for alleviating stress and, in some cases, for bringing about significant personal growth. Of the many meditative techniques that have cropped up since the 1960s, we have chosen to describe the one that put the subject on the map—the Transcendental Meditation (TM) program of Maharishi Mahesh Yogi. The reasons for this choice are that we are personally familiar with TM; it is highly standardized, widely available, and easily learned; its effects go beyond muscular relaxation; and a good deal of scientific research has documented its effects on insomnia and related problems.

Regarding TM and sleep, psychiatrist Harold Bloomfield has written: "Middle-aged patients with complaints of chronic insomnia report improvement in their sleep patterns within the first two or three weeks of meditation. This improvement in their sleep tends to continue until night sedation is no longer necessary, even in previously severe insomnia."

Psychologist Donald E. Miskiman, of the University of Alberta in Canada, studied a group of insomniacs who averaged

75.6 minutes of being awake before falling asleep. Thirty days after taking the TM course the average time of sleep onset dropped to 15.1 minutes!

Many insomniacs who learn TM notice that they sleep for longer periods of time at first. The explanation seems to be that the body compensates for the previous loss of sleep. Within a few weeks, normal sleep patterns tend to resume. Deeper sleep has been reported, as has the need for less total sleep time.

Although improvement seems to come quickly, in many cases insomnia lingers for some time. This might indicate that a certain amount of patience and continued practice is required, or it might indicate that other procedures recommended in this book should also be employed. You shouldn't expect overnight miracles from this or any other technique.

If the TM program does not substantially improve your sleep, it should at least help you cope with sleep loss. In one study, meditators who were subjected to 40 hours of sleep deprivation recovered more quickly than did a control group of nonmeditators, as measured by the amount of compensatory dreaming required once sleeping was resumed. Dr. Miskiman explained the phenomenon this way: "Transcendental Meditation seems to stabilize the sleep-dream cycle by reducing the effect of any disruption to this cycle and thereby restoring the system more quickly to its normal level of functioning."

It should be noted that TM is not done before bed as a way to induce sleep. It is typically practiced for 20-minute periods, morning and afternoon, as a prelude to activity. Experience has shown that if done at bedtime, meditation will probably calm agitated persons enough to enable them to fall asleep, but because of the energy boost it provides, the person might awaken shortly thereafter. Hence, it is not advisable for the evening, as it might further disrupt the sleep/waking cycle. The technique's influence on nighttime sleep seems to be a carryover from the stress-reducing effects of the daytime sessions.

Experiments on physiological changes such as oxygen consumption, heart rate, breath rate, skin resistance, and lactate concentration indicate that the TM technique produces an extraordinarily deep state of rest. TM teachers say that this state penetrates much more deeply than ordinary muscular tension, thus enabling the brain and nervous system to "normalize." In other words, simple relaxation is only one of the technique's advantages.

Studies also show that TM produces an unusually orderly, stable, and coherent style of brain functioning, as indicated by brain-wave patterns. In addition, behavioral studies report enhanced creativity, learning ability, reaction time, academic and job performance, and improvement on self-actualization measures. "Meditators make fewer mistakes, and suffer fewer frustrations," said one researcher, "which should make their heads more carefree when they hit the pillow at night."

If you are interested in learning TM, don't be put off by its Eastern origins, or by the private religious beliefs of its founder, Maharishi Mahesh Yogi, a Hindu monk. The TM technique is a mental one, requiring no changes in life-style, values, or religious and philosophical convictions. It is not incompatible with Western ways, as 30 years of acceptance suggests, and is quite scientific in its approach.

Although the technique is easy to practice, it nevertheless must be learned through private instruction. Its teachers are certified by a large international organization that provides precise instruction and ongoing guidance to meditators. Representatives maintain that no book can teach the technique properly, which is why we have not attempted to do so here.

Although the insistence on private instruction irritates many who believe that the same results can be obtained through written instructions, this premise has not been adequately tested, and TM teachers insist that certain nuances can't be translated to the printed page. They also point out that because you can't ask a book a question, learning meditation from the printed word can be haphazard, incomplete, and even dangerous.

The technique itself revolves around the mental use of sounds called *mantras*. The vibratory frequencies of these sounds, which have been handed down through an ancient tradition, are said to resonate harmoniously with the meditators' nervous systems, bringing about the state of orderly, alert rest described earlier.

During private instruction, the TM teacher assigns a mantra individually, according to certain criteria that he will not divulge. The teacher then guides the student in proper use of the mantra through a series of steps, each of which depends on the student's experiences. Follow-up consists of three evening sessions on consecutive days and unlimited free consultation thereafter.

Your telephone directory should list your local center under Transcendental Meditation. For information and referrals, write to the World Plan Executive Council, 5000 14th St. NW, Washington, DC 20011.

BIOFEEDBACK

Touted by its proponents as a spectacular scientific breakthrough, biofeedback training has captured the attention of researchers and therapists throughout the world. Many see it as a sort of technological panacea with which we will eventually regulate our glandular secretions, control cancer, and even remove warts—all through mind control.

In biofeedback, you are hooked up to equipment that can monitor events in the body—brain waves, heartbeat, blood pressure, skin temperature, muscular tension, stomach acidity, and others depending on the purpose of the session. These events are translated technologically into readily observable signals such as lights, tones, or wavy lines. Once you can, as it were, "see" your heartbeats, or "hear" your brain activity, you have information that can, presumably, help you control those specific functions.

There are five basic steps involved in all biofeedback procedures:

1. A physiological parameter is measured—for example, temperature or heart rate.
2. The measurement is displayed to the person (you), that is, it is fed back.
3. Through trial and error you learn what you must do to change the display.
4. Changes in the correct direction are reinforced by the feedback—you see indications of success.
5. With success, you learn which internal cues are associated with the reinforced changes. Ultimately, you will no longer need the feedback display, but can control the physiological parameter directly.

Biofeedback advocates claimed early on that the procedure would remedy certain ailments—such as migraine headaches, tension, epilepsy, cardiac arrhythmias, and high blood pressure—and subsequent studies suggest that they may have been correct. Some practitioners say they have had dramatic success in treating insomnia. Dr. Thomas Budzynski of the University of Colorado, for example, has devised a training session in which insomniacs are taught to reproduce body-wave and brain-wave patterns associated with the onset of sleep. "With this training," Budzynski reports, "people who had taken four hours to fall asleep were dropping into slumber twice in a 20-minute lab session." He foresees the day when doctors will dispense biofeedback machines instead of sleeping pills.

The most reliable equipment for monitoring and reporting bodily signals is not amenable to home use; it is very expensive and cumbersome, and must be operated by skilled technicians. Other devices—ranging from desktop machines to pen-sized gadgets that measure skin temperature—are available commercially, but they are not always accurate and if you use them on your own you will not have the benefit of a physician or trained technician to guide you. Some biofeedback practitioners will train you in their offices and then provide simple devices with which you can practice at home.

As long as it's properly administered, biofeedback would seem to be a worthwhile approach to investigate. Although not enough research has been done specifically on the effect of biofeedback on sleep, measurable benefits have been gained in related areas, such as controlling hypertension and inducing muscle relaxation. Enough is known about the process, and the techniques have been refined enough over the past decade, that insomniacs need feel no trepidation in trying it out.

If you are inclined to experiment with biofeedback, be sure to obtain your training from a physician or therapist well-versed in the procedure, preferably one associated with a reputable hospital or university—and one who has had experience working with sleep problems.

EXERCISE YOUR WAY TO SLEEP

When Theodore Dreiser was a struggling young writer suffering from insomnia, he got a job as a section hand on the New York Central Railway. After a day of driving spikes and shoveling gravel, he was so exhausted he could hardly stay awake long enough to eat dinner.

You needn't become a manual laborer in order to feel tired at bedtime. But if you lead a sedentary life during the day, it is a good bet that exercise will prove to be a significant aid in attaining better sleep. Research has established that vigorous exercise during the day, or mild exercise at bedtime, increases the amount of Stage IV sleep, the deepest part of the non-REM cycle. "Regular exercise promotes deep sleep," writes sleep researcher Quentin R. Regestein. "Insomniac patients should exercise vigorously and frequently."

Just about every insomniac to whom we suggested increased exercise claimed to have slept better when he or she followed the advice. Several claimed to have overcome the problem entirely. One young man said his insomnia began at the time of an athletic injury in college, three years earlier. The injury ended a promising basketball career, and threw the victim into a state of depression. He attributed his insomnia to the depression, but in fact the sleep problem persisted long after the gloom disappeared and the young man had adjusted to the life of an ex-athlete. Then he began exercising again—more to lose some accumulated poundage than to improve his sleep—and he immediately noticed an improvement in his sleep. He concluded that his body, accustomed to strenuous work all its life, sorely missed the daily workouts that had ended with his injury.

Your body was meant to be used. If you don't move enough, your circulation and breathing can become sluggish. Lactic acid, which has been correlated with stress, accumulates in the blood. Tension builds in the muscles. The brain can even become dull. And you might have trouble sleeping because pent-up energy is keeping your nervous system at a high idle and your muscles are aching to move, not rest.

In addition to providing an outlet for pent-up energy, exercise can charge the nervous system with vitality, activate the all-important endocrine glands, stimulate and strengthen internal organs such as the heart and lungs, and improve mental functioning. In addition, exercise seems to help lift the clouds of boredom, worry, and tension that can contribute to sleep problems. Studies have shown that the hormone epinephrine, a chemical that has been linked with feelings of happiness, doubles in the body after 10 minutes of sustained exercise. This can result in long-lasting pleasurable effects. And, more recent research has shown that exercise stimulates *endorphins*, the body's natural chemicals for alleviating pain; higher levels of endorphins are associated with feelings of well-being.

With the boom in fitness that erupted in the 1970s and was sustained throughout the 1980s, it is now commonplace for doctors to recommend aerobic exercise for their patients regardless of age, especially in cases where the patient does not move around much in the course of his regular routine. Only 15 or 20 minutes of vigorous exercise four times a week will go a long way toward turning most people into fit specimens with a better chance of avoiding cardiovascular disease. And exercise can trigger dramatic changes in people with depression, anxiety, and high levels of tension. One psychiatrist has found that the more people jog the more vividly they dream, and the more their deeper emotions become accessible to their conscious awareness. Such findings should be encouraging to insomniacs who suspect that emotional factors are contributing to their problems.

Furthermore, leg circulation has been found to have an important influence on sleep. Dr. Paul Dudley White, speaking of using the leg muscles, said: "The fatigue produced by it is undoubtedly the best tranquilizer ever made, either by nature or man."

Insomniacs can verify this fact. The next time you have difficulty falling asleep, or when you awaken in the night, notice the feeling in your legs. Often, you will feel a sort of dull sensation or a restlessness, as though your legs want to move even though the rest of you wants to sleep. You might have the urge to massage or stretch your legs. If such signs are present, it is a good bet that leg circulation is playing a role in keeping you awake. Massaging your legs, stretching, or walking around the room may help at the time. But regular exercise is essential.

Of course, jogging is the most popular form of everyday aerobic exercise. But it is not the only way to obtain aerobic benefits. Swimming, bicycling, skipping rope, dancing, pedaling on a stationary bike, or using a treadmill will get your heart and lungs working and give those leg muscles an opportunity to move.

Perhaps the cheapest, easiest, and most accessible form of exercise is plain old walking. If other forms of exercise are incompatible with your way of life, you should at least get into the habit of walking wherever possible instead of relying on conveniences that save time but do little good for your body. Says Dr. Frederick J. Stare of Harvard: "The sedentary businessman should make exercise a part of his daily life. He ought to get into the habit, for instance, of walking instead of taking cabs for short rides. He ought to walk up a flight or two of stairs at the office instead of always taking the elevator."

With respect to sleep, *when* you exercise may be as important as *how* you exercise. Although exercise relaxes the muscles, it can also rev up your body. Exercising late in the evening may speed you up and invigorate you just when you want to slow down. Experts say the best time to work out is early in the morning before breakfast (never immediately after a meal) when the air is fresh and clean. However, insomniacs may find it more sleep-inducing to exercise in the late afternoon or early evening. Some studies have shown that vigorous exercise at that time can increase the percentage of Stages III and IV of sleep.

If you are not used to regular exercise, don't start by entering a marathon. Too much too soon can be dangerous. Start slowly and work your way up gradually to more vigorous levels. Especially if you are over 40, it is a good idea to get a checkup before you begin a regular exercise program. Many doctors recommend having a stress test, which involves running on a treadmill or pedaling on a stationary bike while your heart rate, EKG, blood pressure, and oxygen consumption are monitored.

Getting your body tired with vigorous exercise might be the single best piece of advice an insomniac can receive. It may not be the answer to every person's sleep problem, but it can help.

YOUR JOB AND YOUR SLEEP

Most of us spend about one third of our lives at work. Our experiences there—successes and failures, satisfactions and frustrations, working conditions, relationships with fellow workers—can have a significant effect on our stress levels and therefore our sleep. Here are some things to keep in mind about the vital relationship between those eight hours of work and the eight hours you'd like to sleep.

Two categories of workers have virtually chronic sleep disorders but accept them as "normal" for people in their occupations: shift workers, and those who cross time zones regularly.

In 1989, a new category of insomnia was added to the nomenclature of sleep research: "delayed sleep phase insomnia." This occurs when shift work, for example, disrupts normal sleep/wake schedules and impairs the person's circadian rhythm patterns. Studies have shown that when normal, healthy subjects have their sleep/wake cycles reversed, they begin to have frequent awakenings and can't sustain normal sleep. People who work at night and sleep during the day often suffer severe sleep difficulties that require only a change in schedule to remedy. Nature may not have intended for them to be owls.

The problems of night-shifters are often compounded because their homes are noisy and active just when they are trying to sleep. Perhaps more important, they feel deprived of normal family and social pleasures, so they might further disturb their sleep by trying to remain awake in order to spend more time with their children and spouses. Typically, when weekends and holidays roll around, shift workers try to revert to sleeping at night with everyone else. This further confounds the body's inability to adapt.

Most severely affected are those workers who are called upon to change shifts often. Many industries have their employees rotate day and night shifts. Doctors, nurses, police, firefighters—all are typically called upon to be awake when their bodies think it is time to sleep. The solution? It's a trade-off. Individuals and companies might have to rethink priorities. Perhaps in nonessential areas it might be worth a temporary disruption for the sake of complying with nature's intentions and letting people sleep enough to work more effectively.

Pilots and flight attendants, as well as businesspeople, athletes, and others who pile up frequent-flyer mileage, have to deal with jet lag. As a result of crossing time zones, their usual sleep/wake rhythms are often out of sync with their localities, especially when they fly west to east. The businessman who flies from San Francisco to New York to London, for example, might find himself unable to get to sleep because it is only 5 or 8 P.M. in his body even though his hotel clock reads 2 A.M. It might take days or weeks to readjust. Unfortunately, before that happens the person is likely to be long gone to another time zone, only to have the same problem there.

One proposed solution for those who jet around constantly is to maintain their personal clocks in tune with a single time zone. That is, instead of trying to adapt to each new location, continue to sleep according to the time of your most frequent location, preferably that of home. Although this may hamper a person's social life while traveling and make business meetings more difficult to schedule for everyone's convenience, a decent night's sleep can be worth the price.

Here is a list of other suggestions for overcoming jet lag on isolated journeys:

- When flying east, fly early in the day; when flying west, fly late.
- Four days prior to your trip, begin following this diet regimen: eat high-protein meals the first day, then on the second day eat lightly, favoring liquids, fruit, and salad. Repeat the heavy first-day diet on the third day and the lighter second-day diet on the fourth day, the day of departure.
- Before and during the flight, try to walk and stretch as much as possible.
- In-flight, drink a lot of water and juice; avoid caffeine and alcohol.
- On arrival, adopt local time and routines immediately.

- Get outdoors in the sunlight as much as possible. Exposure to sunlight evidently helps the body to reset its biological clock. (If you must remain indoors, try to arrange the room so that sunlight—or artificial light if necessary—is plentiful.)

Most shift workers and constant travelers are aware of the cause of their sleeplessness. However, when they try to overcome it with sleeping pills, as many do, they compound the problem unnecessarily. Suppose, for example, a San Francisco businesswoman is lying awake at midnight thinking about a 9 A.M. meeting. Anxious about being tired in the morning, she pops a pill and starts the kind of dependency pattern we described in chapter 3.

Similarly, the night worker who wants to be able to get to sleep at the same time as his family on Saturday night so he can spend Sunday with them may also resort to pills. Or, in his determination to fall asleep, he struggles and strains when he ought to be relaxing. In the case of the pill, he may, indeed, get to sleep, but he is not likely to feel at his best in the morning. And if he tries too strenuously to fall asleep, the frustration will only keep him awake and make him an intolerable grouch the next day, just when he wants to enjoy his family.

Fitting Work Hours to Sleep Needs

If possible, arrange your working hours to fit your sleep needs. This is not always easy to do, of course, but, depending on your position, you will be surprised at how easy it might be to rearrange your schedule. Bill Forman is a salesman for a large manufacturing company. Every morning he would awaken at about 4, perfectly refreshed. However, he needed a good, solid nap in the afternoon or he would be foggy and dull. Bill did not feel right taking a nap during working hours, so he just trudged through as best he could, but his performance after lunch did not measure up to his morning standards. Finally, the situation became unbearable.

Forman and his boss had a long talk, the upshot of which was that the salesman scheduled all his meetings with customers between 9 A.M. and 1 P.M. and was allowed to do all his paperwork whenever convenient. He could do his paperwork very early in the morning and nap in the afternoon. His productivity and happiness rose markedly.

When you *don't* work is as important as when you do. It is essential to end your work day well in advance of bedtime. You should ease into sleep, not crash into it. Many busy executives have difficulty getting to sleep at night for the simple reason that they keep on working until right before they turn out the lights. One corporate vice president, Jane Bunker, would take work home every night. She would not only read reports in bed but would even listen to tapes of business conferences while washing up and brushing her teeth. Needless to say, it took her so long to fall asleep that she kept a vial of sleeping pills handy on her night table.

Only the onset of ulcers got Bunker to reevaluate her habits. The first thing the doctor told her was to leave her work at the office. Within a few weeks, she was sleeping relatively easily and did not refill her sleeping-pill prescription.

Fill the pre-bed hours with something pleasant, soothing, and unstrained. Take your spouse or a good book to bed with you, not your work.

Pacing yourself properly is also important. Your job should have breaks built into it as well as decent vacation opportunities. Many ambitious people have driven themselves to success only to discover they are too tired or too sick to enjoy it. A hard day's work can either make you sleep like a baby or keep you tossing and turning all night. According to Dr. Hans Selye, the renowned expert on stress, "A stressful activity which has come to a definite stop prepares you for rest and sleep; but one which sets up self-maintaining tensions keeps you awake."

Dr. Selye offered these points of vocational advice for insomniacs:

"Do not let yourself get carried away and keyed up more than is necessary to acquire the momentum for the best performance.

"Keep in mind that the hormones produced during acute stress are meant to alarm you and key you up for peak accomplishments. They tend to combat sleep.

"Try not to overwork any one part of your body or mind disproportionately by repeating the same actions to exhaustion. Be especially careful to avoid the senseless repetition of the same task when you are already exhausted."

Your work should be enjoyable. Spending eight or more hours a day wishing you were somewhere else is not conducive to sleep. You will seethe inside, the tension will build, and you will end up spending half your nights wallowing in anger and bitterness, mentally telling off everyone from your boss to your clients and colleagues to your high-school guidance counselor. It is not asking too much of life to work at a job that you like, especially if not doing so prevents you from obtaining a good night's sleep.

This does not mean eliminating challenges and problems. That would not only make for a dull life, it could also keep you up at night. Boredom and monotony can be stressful; ruts are also a major source of insomnia. The mysterious "weekend insomniacs" who only have sleep problems when they are not working are quite likely bored. They lack an outlet for their energy, which, going unreleased, keeps them wired at night.

Keep happily busy, therefore, with challenging, constructive work and hobbies and social activities you enjoy. Mary Platt, a Boston housewife, is a good example of an insomniac who solved her problem that way. Mary had been a sound sleeper until her three children were grown and living away from home. Then she suddenly couldn't sleep. After it was determined that medical factors were not responsible, her doctor began to suspect that Mrs. Platt was simply bored and feeling useless. As a result, he advised her to get involved in community activities and resume former hobbies such as playing the piano. She did, and her sleep was soon restored to normal.

DAYTIME NAPS FOR NIGHTTIME SLEEP

The eccentric genius Salvador Dali used to sit in a chair holding a spoon loosely between his fingers. On the floor beneath the dangling spoon he would place a tin plate. Then he would close his eyes. When sleep came, the spoon would fall, and the clatter of metal would jolt the artist awake. Dali claimed he was completely refreshed after such a short period of sleep.

Less bizarre but nonetheless unusual was Eleanor Roosevelt's habit of stealing a furtive one-minute snooze while sitting perfectly upright at a dinner party. She was also said to nap regularly on speakers' platforms, always awakening just before she was introduced.

It might take some time and luck before you gain the napping proficiency of a Dali or Mrs. Roosevelt, but acquiring the skill might do more for your insomnia than a bookful of medical advice. In many cases, a nap can help alleviate the aftermath of a fitful night, and may also help prevent further trouble the next night.

The advisability of napping for insomniacs is a disputed point. Some experts recommend it, whereas others are unequivocally opposed to it and consider napping detrimental to evening slumber. Anti-nap physicians say that irregular daytime naps can lead to erratic sleep at night. They prefer patients to establish a regular sleep rhythm, going to sleep at approximately the same time every night. Usually, they advocate eliminating naps, although some will permit them if they are taken as a routine at the same time every day.

From all indications, napping is an individual matter,

good for some insomniacs, not so good for others. If you have initial insomnia (difficulty falling asleep), and are accustomed to napping during the day, you might do well to eliminate the naps long enough to see if they are, in fact, interfering with your sleep. During this experiment, go to bed at the same time every night.

Napping might be good if yours is the type of insomnia that awakens you prematurely and unrefreshed. Conceivably, your internal rhythms are better suited to early rising with a compensatory 40 winks during the day than to the standard eight solid hours at night. One insomniac we know, who had tried a number of remedies to no avail, finally found that a good nap after lunch was all he needed.

"I used to get up at dawn unable to fall back to sleep," he said. "I was okay for a few hours but then I would be overcome by fatigue and I'd drag through the rest of the day. Often I would collapse in bed, exhausted but unable to sleep through the whole night. Finally, in desperation, I cut my lunch hour short and added a nap. If I oversleep, my boss lets me make up the time later on."

The widespread belief that an afternoon nap will make you too alert to fall asleep at night is not true for everyone. Overexhaustion can actually hinder natural sleep. Dr. Philip Tiller of the Louisiana State School of Medicine conducted an experiment with several hundred women who had complained of being nervous, fatigued, and generally run down. They each took a one- or two-hour nap every afternoon. Dr. Tiller then determined that the naps helped the women sleep better at night. About two thirds of the women reported a significant decrease in other symptoms as well.

Some believe that naps shorter than two hours are not restful since the body does not have time to go through the entire non-REM and REM cycle. This has been disputed. "You don't need certain amounts of REM or slow-wave [Stage IV] sleep to function effectively," stated one scientist. "This idea prevailed until the late 1950s and '60s. But it has been dis-proven." In fact, Dr. Timothy Roehrs of the Henry Ford Hospital in Detroit says that afternoon naps usually consist of a high degree of deep non-REM sleep, which is why short naps, like small diamonds, can pack a lot of value.

If you decide to tune out for a few minutes in the middle of the day, don't feel guilty. You will be in good company. Most cultures have institutionalized rest periods of greater length than our own lunch and coffee breaks, and they tend to be more tranquil as well. In Europe, most everything closes for two or three hours at midday, to provide not only a lei-surely lunch break but a comfortable siesta.

History's artful nappers include such high achievers as Thomas Edison (who slept for five hours at night and cat-napped as needed), General Douglas MacArthur, Napoleon, and presidents Teddy Roosevelt, Harry S Truman, Dwight D. Eisenhower, John F. Kennedy, and Lyndon B. Johnson. Wrote Winston Churchill in *The Gathering Storm:* "I always went to bed at least for one hour as early as possible in the afternoon and exploited to the full my happy gift of falling almost imme-diately to sleep. By this means I was able to press a day and a half's work into one. Nature had not intended mankind to work from eight in the morning until midnight without the refreshment of blessed oblivion, which, even if it lasts only twenty minutes, is sufficient to renew all vital forces."

Among contemporary artful nappers are Henry Kissinger, who was known to fall asleep sitting upright on a plane; Bar-bara Walters, who says she can fall asleep in any chair; and Robert Fulghum, who in 1989 had two books on the best-seller list at the same time (*All I Really Need to Know I Learned in Kindergarten* and *It Was on Fire When I Lay Down on It*). "I don't care if people make fun of me for it," he says. "Once a day I lie down on my back and calm down and I'm going to live to be an old man because of that."

One reason napping can improve normal sleep is that it

can help your day go better, thus leaving you with fewer cares at night. Several studies suggest that nappers tend to be more alert, be less tense, and score better on performance tests than their non-napping counterparts. Dr. Charles Fisher, a New York psychoanalyst who has researched sleep for some twenty-five years, says: "We still don't know, scientifically, why so short a sleep—ten minutes, one minute—can be refreshing to many people. It could be that it stops conscious thought processes, and in this way relieves anxiety. Or, as has been found, nondreaming sleep helps the problem-solving mechanism."

Of course, taking a snooze during the day might not be compatible with your job. Said the chairman of a major firm when asked how he would feel if an employee nodded out on company time, "I would figure he needed the rest of the afternoon off, probably the next morning, and maybe a long time after that." Nevertheless, a little logic and a sincere attitude might be enough to convince your boss of the advantages of letting you tune out for a while during office hours.

You needn't have a proper bedroom to nap in. A sofa, a carpeted floor, even a comfortable chair will do. Some people keep a foldaway cot or foam-rubber pad in their offices along with a blanket and pillow. Many companies have infirmaries with cots that employees are welcome to use.

If you have the opportunity to nap, the best time is said to be just after lunch, the traditional siesta time. Certainly, napping at that hour is less likely to disturb your nighttime sleep than snoozing at, say, 6 or 7 P.M. If you decide to experiment with napping, settle on a convenient time and take your nap at that same time every day. Regularity is important. Studies indicate that irregular nappers tend to be groggy, irritable, and disoriented after their nap—and, they often have trouble sleeping at night.

If you've set a napping schedule, try to find time to lie down at the predetermined hour every day, even if you do not feel sleepy at the time. Give yourself at least fifteen minutes. Even if you don't fall asleep, you will probably feel remarkably refreshed from just lying there. If anyone objects to your snoozing when there is work to be done and problems to solve, you might point out that many great scientific discoveries (for example, the structure of the benzine molecule) and artistic creations (Coleridge's "Kubla Khan") were conceived during sleep. Just tell them you're sleeping on it.

CHAPTER 6

Eat Right to Sleep Tight

Your foods shall be your remedies, and your remedies shall be your foods.

HIPPOCRATES

A 1927 magazine advertisement promised: "Tonight, you can get eight hours of solid sleep—*without the use of drugs.* Tomorrow, you should awaken abounding with new-found vigor." The product being promoted was a new cereal beverage named Ovaltine, which the ad said would give you "sound, restful sleep in a *natural* way."

The efficacy of Ovaltine as a sleep remedy aside, those early ad writers were attuned to a logic that seems to have escaped most modern physicians: since sleep is such a fundamental biochemical phenomenon, it is doubtless affected by what we eat and drink. Anyone who has ever tossed and turned to the rumbling of too much pizza and ice cream can certainly testify to that. Given the typical American diet, it is not inconceivable that many sleep problems are caused by metabolic imbalances resulting from wrong eating habits. Even if diet as such is not the *cause*, it can certainly be a contributing factor and a potential aspect of a cure. Nutrition should be a vital consideration in any natural treatment regimen.

In our search for nutritional approaches to sleep problems, we had to investigate sources outside the realm of orthodox medicine since nutrition is not even a required subject in most medical schools and most doctors undervalue diet as a form of treatment. Nevertheless, we found that legitimate nutritional expertise is plentiful. There are a number of books and a plethora of dieticians, nutritionists, and holistic health practitioners who use diet as a key component of their treatments. There is even an entire discipline called *orthomolecular psychiatry* whose adherents use large doses of vitamins and dietary regimens to the virtual exclusion of pharmaceuticals and standard psychotherapeutic procedures.

In short, nutritional information is widely available—so much so that it is just as easy to find contradictions, fanaticism, and dubious claims as it is to find prudent advice. One must tread carefully and analytically before deciding on a change in diet. Indeed, too rapid or drastic a change, even in the right direction, can be dangerous. Nevertheless, sensibly approached, what you do at the table might be the key to changing what happens in bed.

A VISIT TO A NUTRITIONIST

We wanted to submit ourselves to a nutritional regimen under the supervision of an expert to see how it affected our sleep. We selected Samuel ("Sy") Bursuk, a consulting health educator and nutritionist for the North Nassau Mental Health Center on Long Island, because he had a history of sleep problems himself, which he claimed to have cured through nutrition.

Well-tanned and sporting an engaging smile, Bursuk looked as if he might be more at home in Southern California or Florida than the New York City suburb where he works. He described his insomnia, which began during a stressful period of his life: "I was restless; I awakened unrefreshed. At the height of my illness, sleep was completely broken. Rarely did I get more than 2 hours of real sleep a night. I would lie in bed for as long as 16 hours a day with my eyes closed, but not sleeping. This lasted nine months or a year."

During that period, Bursuk visited two psychiatrists, an internist, an endocrinologist, and a psychotherapist. Heavily drugged by those experts with phenothiazine and other antipsychotic drugs, including some for sleep, he was eventually hospitalized by what he now calls an overdose. His condition turned around when, on the advice of a friend, he visited a doctor with an orientation toward nutrition. The physician took a comprehensive medical history, a battery of biochemical blood tests, and a six-hour glucose-tolerance test. On the basis of his findings, he prescribed a diet and put Bursuk on a program of supplemental vitamins and minerals.

The change in Bursuk's sleeping pattern was remarkable. "I was sleeping less, and sleeping better," he says. "I would wake up and bounce out of bed." Attributing the change in his condition to a rebalancing of his body chemistry, achieved primarily through nutritional means, he decided to change professions from engineering to health.

Now, as a nutritional consultant to doctors and dentists, he brings to his work the sort of compassion that only a former sufferer can. Through an analysis of his clients' eating patterns, their responses to a questionnaire, and optional laboratory tests, Bursuk recommends a nutritional program. With insomniacs, the first thing he does is to steer his clients away from thinking of their insomnia as a disease. "Don't isolate the sleep mechanism," he warns. "Insomnia is a sign, not a disease." When people come to him with chronic sleep problems, he invariably discovers other, more serious problems that suggest a general physiological imbalance.

"The primary cause of insomnia," Bursuk believes, "is faulty digestion. That leads to deficiencies of vitamins, minerals, and enzymes." He views the human organism as a biochemical machine run by metabolism. If you put junk into it, you will get faulty performance, just as you would if you put kerosene into your car instead of gas. Conversely, he says, "If you put in what nature intended, the body is self-balancing, self-cleansing, and self-healing. When the body is in balance, or homeostasis, it becomes disease-resistant."

Overcoming insomnia through nutrition is not an overnight process, Bursuk cautions. He recalls that in his own case the sleep mechanism was the last thing to normalize. And, he warns, treating physical problems through nutrition differs from the kind of treatment we are used to—unlike injections or surgery, it can't be done for you or to you. It requires discipline. Without that, you are not likely to follow the program as prescribed and you will fall back into old eating habits before your body can restore its equilibrium. That is a point well worth remembering if you choose to change your diet in hope of improving your sleep.

Because we thought that Bursuk's status as a formerly severe insomniac would give him a level of insight that another nutritionist might lack, we decided that one of us should become a client of his. Here is the report:

"During my initial consultation, I filled out a lengthy questionnaire and answered Sy's questions for about an hour. For the next two weeks, as instructed, I kept a running list of everything I ate, and I took my pulse rate on arising, before and after meals, and before bed. And every morning I tested my urine for a deficiency in hydrochloric acid. A hair test designed to diagnose mineral deficiencies was done later by a laboratory.

"A week after the results were in, Sy handed me a large, heavy paper bag. 'Here are your supplements,' he said. Eleven jars! I was to take them after each meal in different combinations: eleven in the morning, eight after lunch, and thirteen after dinner. The list included: a high-potency multivitamin that contained just about everything you can think of;

vitamins A, D, C, and E; bone meal, a calcium supplement; pantothenic acid; wheat germ oil; a digestive enzyme; and enzymes for the liver, pancreas, and adrenal glands.

"Sy felt that hypoglycemia (low blood sugar) was a major factor in my sleep problems. In fact, I had been diagnosed hypoglycemic two years earlier, and while following the prescribed diet at the time, my sleep had improved. Recently, however, I'd gotten careless and found my sleep once again disturbed.

"I was given a list of allowed foods and forbidden foods. The former consisted of good, healthy items with an emphasis on fresh fruits and vegetables, and protein—non–red-meat sources preferred. In the forbidden category were all the items I love to junk on and feel guilty about afterward, especially sugar.

"In fact, the diet was not difficult to adhere to. The hardest part of Sy's regimen was taking the supplements. Remembering to take them was the first problem. Then I had to overcome the annoyance of the process itself—opening all those little jars and removing one or two tablets, while simultaneously checking the list to make sure I hadn't forgotten one, or taken too many of another, or taken the lunchtime combination instead of the dinner. It seemed incredibly tedious. Perhaps more significantly, I calculated that if I continued taking the supplements in that dosage I would spend well over $700 a year on vitamins and minerals. That's enough to make you lose sleep—or at least convince yourself that you don't need supplements.

"I wondered if Sy and other health-food advocates don't become a tad overzealous about prescribing supplements. Sy contended, and most of his colleagues concur, that supplements would be unnecessary if we could eat the way nature intended. But food that is processed, preserved, packaged, and otherwise tampered with invariably loses vital nutrients. In addition, he told me, most of us have damaged our digestive systems through years of bad habits. Thus, our bodies are unable adequately to assimilate what we put into them.

"I followed Sy's program as closely as I could. I noticed some changes rather quickly—an increase of physical strength, some extra vitality, perhaps less fatigue during the day. Not all the changes were pleasant, however. I had some indigestion immediately after eating and taking the supplements. And my sleep did not improve. In fact, on some nights it was worse—I awakened with stomach cramps. Sy was not surprised. He attributed this to what he called 'the healing crisis.' Because of improper digestion, he explained, toxins had accumulated in my system. The enzymes speed up the eliminative process, and the toxins start to be flushed out through the bloodstream. During the period of adaptation, indigestion, sluggishness, or perhaps moodiness can result temporarily. Sy adjusted my regimen to slow down the eliminative process. The symptoms abated, and I soon resumed the original program. This time there were no side effects.

"After four months of relatively faithful adherence to my diet, I concluded that it was probably—along with meditation and exercise—among the most significant things I had done for my sleep problems. I woke up less frequently and, when I did wake up, I found it easier to fall back to sleep. By contrast, when I cheated on my diet I did not sleep as well. The correlation was as clear as day. If I went on a sugar binge, for example, or if I neglected to eat enough protein, or if I went too long without eating, I reverted back to my previous difficulties."

Our conclusion is that nutrition can be an important line of defense for insomniacs. Ideally, you should work out a regimen in consultation with an expert, since self-prescribed programs are bound to be less precise, less reliable, and less safe. But since professional help is too costly for some and not easily available to others, we combed the nutritional bookshelves for anything that was relevant to sleep and insomnia, trying to steer clear of faddists and fanatics. We found certain points reiterated over and over again. These are recounted in the following sections.

EXTRACT YOUR SWEET TOOTH

Things sweet to taste prove in digestion sour.
SHAKESPEARE, *Richard II*

An insomniac stockbroker we know used to fall asleep all right but would wake up five or six hours later feeling as if his nervous system was "one big, twanging guitar string." Though he was so tired he felt immobile, he would feel a buzz of activity inside. Thoughts raced through his mind as if he were in the midst of a crisis, only they were all disconnected, unrealistic, and irrelevant. His heart pounded furiously. Yet he felt exhausted, unable to get out of bed. He wanted to sleep more.

Sometimes the broker would lie in this netherworld of nonsleep and nonwaking for an hour or more before trudging through his morning routine. During the day, he was alternatively depressed and elated, speedy and lethargic, pleasant and gloomy. The pattern continued until a doctor asked about his late-night eating habits. On hearing that the sufferer was fond of sugary snacks, the doctor suggested a blood test. Sure enough, the diagnosis was an imbalance of blood sugar. A change in diet resulted in dramatic improvement.

Whether your insomnia is like the stockbroker's, or you can't fall asleep at all, your blood sugar may be a factor. If you are an occasional insomniac, chances are the nights that you have difficulty are the very nights that you eat sweets or starches in abundance. Check your diet chart and see.

We are a nation of sugar junkies. According to Drs. Emanuel Cheraskin and William Ringsdorf, Jr., professors of oral medicine at the University of Alabama, "The American eats more candy than eggs; drinks more soft drinks than milk; and downs as much sugar as the combined intake of eggs, all fruits, potatoes, all other vegetables, and whole grain cereals."

Even the conservative *Journal of the American Medical Association* stated that sugar contributes to heart and gall bladder disease, appendicitis, diverticulosis, varicose veins, hiatal hernia, and cancer of the large intestine, as well as insomnia.

Perhaps the most common sugar syndrome is *hypoglycemia*. Dr. Carlton Fredericks, former president of the International Academy of Preventive Medicine, once estimated that there are at least 20 million hypoglycemics in the United States. It is a good bet that most Americans display the classic symptoms of hypoglycemia from time to time even if their conditions are not so severe as to be revealed in a laboratory. So the information in this section might be useful to anyone looking for ways to improve his or her sleep, particularly if you consume too much sugar.

The sugar you consume, and the starches that the body turns quickly into sugar, stimulate the pancreas to secrete insulin, the hormone that transforms sugar and other foods into usable glucose. Too much sugar causes an overproduction of insulin, which in turn burns up not only the sugar you have eaten but some of your reserves of blood sugar as well. This leaves you with too little glucose in the bloodstream, and glucose is the brain's fuel. When it does not get enough glucose from the bloodstream, the brain slows down and the person becomes extremely tired. Normal sleep patterns can be disturbed because the body reacts to the shortage of glucose by going into an emergency state. This speeds up certain of your systems, notably the secretion of emergency hormones in the adrenal and other endocrine glands, and that process interferes with sleep.

The usual pattern of low-blood-sugar victims is to have a rush of energy immediately after eating sugar or starch (when the insulin is stirred to overaction), only to have that episode followed by fatigue, irritability, and possibly dizziness when the sugar level drops below normal. In severe cases, the symptoms can include vertigo, headaches, cramps, tremors, blurred vision, and cold sweats.

Typically, hypoglycemics experience radical shifts of energy and mood—even during the night, which is why they might awaken frequently, bug-eyed and wired for action. In the long run, the abused pancreas stops working correctly and the symptoms become chronic.

If any of this sounds familiar, and especially if you have an active sweet tooth, you should check out whether you have hypoglycemia. Your doctor may scoff at the mention of the word. The symptoms are so commonplace, and nutrition is so widely ignored, that dozens of other explanations also sound plausible. It is not uncommon to run across people who go from doctor to doctor being told that they have some psychological disorder or just "nervous tension," only to find out one day that they have low blood sugar.

Find a doctor that is sympathetic to your theory and have him administer the glucose-tolerance test. It will either eliminate hypoglycemia as a possibility, or it will give you sound clinical evidence that a change in diet is necessary.

The only way to treat hypoglycemia is through diet, and that, ideally, should be adjusted to your individual circumstances—previous habits, taste, weight, and other factors should be considered. However, low-blood-sugar diets all have certain features in common. Even in the absence of a definitive diagnosis, it can't hurt to follow these guidelines to see if your sleep improves.

- Avoid all sugars and sweets. Yes, that means pies, pastries, cookies, candies, sugared breakfast cereals, and other favorite junk snacks.
- Eliminate coffee, tea, and other caffeine-containing beverages. Needless to say, this is important advice for all insomniacs, low blood sugar or not. We will elaborate on caffeine later on.

- Avoid alcohol.

- Reduce your intake of starches—rice, spaghetti, corn, and potatoes (one or two baked potatoes a week are usually permitted). Limit your bread intake to no more than one slice of whole grain bread per meal (no white bread), toasted if possible. Limit peas, lima beans, baked beans, and cereals.

- Reduce consumption of dried fruits such as dates and raisins.

- Eat a lot of protein. It metabolizes slowly and will not induce radical shifts of insulin secretion. In addition to meat and dairy products, nuts, legumes, soybeans, and avocados are excellent sources of protein.

- Keep the size of your meals moderate and snack in between. This is the key factor in regulating blood sugar: frequent meals keep the sugar level evenly distributed throughout the day. Two hours after a main meal, and once an hour thereafter have a glass of fruit juice, a glass of milk, a few nuts, a slice of cheese, or some yogurt. It is probably better to favor protein snacks over the fruits, but seek a proportion that is comfortable and satisfying.

Dr. Carey Reams, a well-respected biophysicist and naturopathic physician, has his patients eat fruits and starches only before two in the afternoon. "Your body needs energy earlier in the day, not toward evening and bedtime. If starchy foods and fruits are eaten after 2 P.M. the energy that's released is not completely used and the sugar builds up in the bloodstream."

If you ever awaken in the middle of the night feeling something similar to the insomniac we described at the beginning of this section, it is quite possible that your blood sugar has gone haywire. Take a slice of cheese or a glass of milk. Half a cup of cottage cheese is good if milk or hard cheese is difficult for you to digest. The added protein might even out the sugar level and allow you to fall back to sleep more easily.

If you have difficulty giving up sugar entirely, try this plan: Cut back, gradually at first, by avoiding sugary and starchy snacks when possible. Eat fruit instead, or nibble on some of the alternatives we mentioned. Then eliminate sugar from your meals, and be vigilant about the ingredients of foods purchased in stores and restaurants, because a great deal of sugar is consumed unknowingly. Soon you will find that you crave sugar less and less, especially if you follow the other basic points of good nutrition.

The following nutritional facts should help you lean toward healthy snacks instead of the sugary or starchy kind: Eating an ounce of sunflower seeds instead of an ounce of potato chips will, in addition to keeping your sugar level moderate, provide you with 4 times as much protein, 4 times as much iron, 3 times as much calcium, 9 times as much thiamine, 3 times as much riboflavin, 14 times as much vitamin A, and twice as much fiber.

If you cut down on sweets, you're more likely to have sweet dreams.

BREAK THE COFFEE-BREAK HABIT

In most parts of the world, coffee is consumed more frequently than any other beverage. Each day Americans consume more than 400 millions cups of coffee, and coffee—in fact all caffeine products, including chocolate, cola, and tea— tends to disturb sleep through its stimulating effects. Caffeine works because it stimulates the adrenal glands to produce hormones that tell the liver to rush glucose into the bloodstream. Hence, a lot of people can't get to sleep because they are so "perked up."

It's a safe bet that a large number of chronic insomniacs could be cured by simply giving up caffeine. Many of them don't even realize how much of the substance they consume, since they don't keep track of their coffee intake and may not even realize that the cokes they gulp down contain caffeine.

The case against caffeine has been studied experimentally, always with reinforcing results: sleep time decreases and the number of awakenings increases when coffee is consumed near bedtime. In a thirteen-night study at the sleep disorders center at Baylor University, eighteen young adult men were given different doses of caffeine a half hour before bed. The researchers found that the equivalent of one cup of regular coffee seemed to have little or no effect on sleep. The two-cup equivalent had its greatest effects early in the night (it took longer to fall asleep, and subjects had less of Stages III and IV). And the four-cup equivalent, needless to say, affected all measures of sleep in large magnitude. Decaffeinated coffee had no effect on sleep.

The researchers postulated that "caffeine somehow exerts its effects on sleep through alterations in brain metabolites." They also postulated that middle-aged and elderly persons might be more sensitive to caffeine than the young adults tested.

According to Dr. Quentin Regestein: "The peak of stimulating action may occur two to four hours after ingestion of caffeine, and the duration of the action lasts from two to seven hours. Coffee drunk hours previously may arouse the patient at bedtime. Insomniac patients frequently resort to [caffeine] to overcome fatigue, and this can result in a vicious cycle of caffeine abuse and sleeplessness."

The best bet, of course, would be to give up caffeine entirely. Next best would be to confine your intake to the morning hours. Naturally, you could consume decaffeinated coffee or tea, or one of the natural grain beverages such as Postum, Pero, or Cafix available at health-food stores. These might take some getting used to if you are a coffee buff. Herbal teas, of course, are a healthy, caffeine-free alternative for those who like warm drinks. In fact, some contain sleep-promoting herbs, which will be discussed more in another chapter.

SOME SALTY ADVICE

The next time you are about to shower your food with table salt, consider this: In excessive concentrations, salt acts as a stimulant to the nervous system. It raises the blood pressure by increasing the accumulation of fluids, and it interferes with the elimination of certain waste products of metabolism. Salt can aggravate insomnia.

Dr. Michael M. Miller of St. Elizabeth's Hospital in Washington, D.C., found that insomniacs whose salt intake was reduced were able to fall asleep within 15 minutes after getting to bed. Most slept through the night. Dr. Miller then restored the salt to thirteen of the twenty-five patients' diets without their knowledge. Within a few days, he reports, ten of them had relapses and could not sleep.

Although the data linking salt and insomnia is by no means sufficient, cutting down your intake would seem a sensible thing to do. Most health experts are opposed to high salt intake for other reasons, principally the deleterious effect of sodium on blood pressure. Your body can certainly do without it. Dr. Mary S. Rose, author of *Foundations of Nutrition,* writes: "The amount of sodium chloride taken in the form of common salt is far in excess of human requirements for sodium and chlorine."

Persons who reduce their salt intake commonly report that their food tastes too bland. Robert Rodale, publisher of *Prevention* magazine, offers this advice: "Go easy on the salt for a week or two, and your desire for that salty taste will decrease. Only for the first ten days or so of the low-salt regimen will you miss that flavor. Then your taste buds will adjust, and you'll enjoy your food just as much even though you're skipping all that sodium, which can raise your blood pressure and do other harmful things."

To be sure you're getting enough sodium in your diet when cutting down on salt, try to eat foods that are high in natural mineral salts—uncooked fruits and vegetables, nuts, and seeds.

CALCIUM

"Calcium can be as soothing as a mother, as relaxing as a sedative, and as life-saving as an oxygen tent," wrote food expert Adelle Davis. "A calcium deficiency often shows itself by insomnia. The harm done by sleeping pills, to say nothing of the thousands of dollars spent annually on them, could largely be avoided if the calcium intake were adequate. Since milk is our richest source of calcium, warm milk drinks taken before retiring have been advertised for relief from insomnia. . . . For the person whose tissues are starved for calcium, however, the amount in a milk drink is a mere drop in the bucket. I usually tell persons whose insomnia is severe to take temporarily two or three calcium tablets with a milk drink before retiring, and to keep both milk and the tablets on a bedside table and take more every hour if wakefulness persists."

According to Dr. H. C. Sherman of Columbia University, 50 percent of the American people are starving for calcium. Even if exaggerated, that fact could go a long way toward explaining the mass insomnia in the United States. Calcium has a calming effect on the nervous system. When deficient in this natural sedative, a person is likely to be tense, grouchy, hyperactive, and overly fatigued. Calcium is also said to be important for the proper functioning of the sleep center in the brain.

How can we be low on calcium when we ingest so much milk, eggs, and other calcium-rich foods? The answer has to do with stress—the same stress that, in other ways, contributes to insomnia. Tension and pressure produce high concentrations of lactic acid in the blood. This acid tends to "bind" the calcium, making it difficult to assimilate.

A quart of milk fortified with a half cup of powdered milk will give you two grams of calcium—the minimum daily amount that Adelle Davis recommended for insomniacs. Cultured buttermilk made from skim milk is said to be an excellent source of calcium, since the acid it contains helps predigest the calcium for easy absorption into the bloodstream.

For the sleepless, Davis suggests four glasses of buttermilk daily, along with generous servings of yogurt.

Other calcium-rich foods to keep around the house: cheese and other dairy products, eggs, figs, oranges, almonds, calcium-rich vegetables such as cauliflower and broccoli, soybeans, turnip greens, and blackstrap molasses. Eskimos, who reportedly sleep like babes despite their unfavorable weather conditions, obtain calcium by consuming large amounts of powdered animal bone. You can purchase bone meal in tablet or powder form at a health-food store.

Calcium deficiencies are often compounded by a deficiency of magnesium, which is important for calcium absorption. According to food experts, our average daily intake of magnesium is about half the adult requirement. If you consume lots of white flour, sugar, or alcohol (even in small amounts) you are likely to be deficient in this important mineral.

Food containing high amounts of magnesium are sea salt, kelp, seeds of all kinds, nuts, beets, spinach, dates, and prunes. You might wish to add magnesium supplements to your diet. In fact, some of the better supplement manufacturers have products that combine calcium and magnesium for maximum absorption.

THE B VITAMINS

One of the founders of orthomolecular psychiatry, Dr. Allan Cott, told us of a study in which subjects who were given 3,000 milligrams of vitamin B_3 (niacinamide) a day recorded a 40 percent increase in REM sleep. He also claimed to have treated many hyperactive children with large doses of niacinamide and found, as a side effect, that they slept better. Dr. Cott explains: "Niacinamide is found in research to enter the biochemical pathway that ends up raising the serotonin level." (Serotonin, as we shall see, is a neurotransmitter associated with the regulation of the sleep mechanism in the brain.) Fifty milligrams of B_3 three times daily has been suggested by orthomolecular psychiatrists to insure better sleep.

Another B vitamin, B_6 (pyridoxine), or the lack of it, has been associated with a host of maladies, including insomnia. According to Dr. Richard W. Vilter, author of *Modern Nutrition in Health and Disease*, persons suffering pyridoxine deficiencies will tend to lose weight and to be apathetic, irritable, and chronically sleepy. Vitamin B_6 is known to have a sedative effect on the nerves, and has been used successfully to treat St. Vitus's dance, palsy, and epilepsy. It also seems necessary for the normal functioning of the brain, and is essential for maintaining the proper level of magnesium in the blood, which, as we have seen, is important for assuring proper calcium absorption.

Of special relevance to insomniacs is the fact that when B_6 is deficient, the amino acid l-tryptophan is not used properly by the body. L-tryptophan is the focal point of promising research on sleep and is discussed later in this chapter.

Many scientists maintain that almost every American is lacking in B_6, although the requirement varies among individuals and families. For example, families in which several members have had diabetes or epilepsy tend to need larger amounts of B_6. Women taking birth control pills are often seriously deficient. And, according to Dr. Ronald Searcy, the amount of B_6 in your system tends to decrease dramatically with age. With these facts in mind, you might have your doctor administer the simple urine test for determining B_6 deficiencies.

Dr. Paul Gyorgy of the University of Pennsylvania suggests B_6 supplements of 25 milligrams daily to prevent insomnia and similar nervous disorders. Others recommend 50 milligrams daily. If you decide to use a supplement, start small and build up only if necessary.

Pantothenic acid, another B vitamin, is needed for the proper functioning of every cell in the body. Neither sugar nor fat can be converted into energy without it. It is also a key nutrient for the functioning of the adrenal glands, and is correlated with allergies and hypoglycemia. From our previous discussions, therefore, it is easy to see why pantothenic acid would be a key factor in sleep.

Experiments by Dr. E. P. Ralli of New York University College of Medicine suggest that pantothenic acid is never toxic, and that it can protect the body from numerous kinds of stress. A daily supplement of 100 milligrams might be a wise addition to an anti-insomnia regime.

Psychiatrists report that vitamin B_{12} treatments have been helpful in treating depression and insomnia. You may comfortably take supplements of 25 milligrams daily. To determine whether you have a serious deficiency of B_{12}, ask your physician to give you a "serum B_{12} test."

The B vitamin inositol has also been used as a natural sleep-aid. It can be purchased in jars of 100 tablets of 650 milligrams each. Try taking two before bed.

Here is a list of foods that are rich in all the B vitamins: liver and other organ meats; whole grains; wheat germ; walnuts; peanuts; bananas; sunflower seeds; blackstrap molasses. The most concentrated source is brewer's yeast, which may be obtained in tablet form or as a powder. (It tastes awful to most people at first, but they quickly get used to it mixed with fruit juice or milk, baked in bread, or sprinkled over cereal.)

A WORD ON SUPPLEMENTS

If, after taking vitamins and minerals for a while, your sleep improves, you might want to start gradually cutting back on the supplements. If you eat right and live right, you may not need more than a good multivitamin. However, in moderation, supplements providing key nutrients such as calcium and the B vitamins can only help. You decide the best strategy. If you decide to take supplements, take them after meals, and spread out the dosage evenly throughout the day, to assure proper absorption.

Ideally, you should consult a qualified nutritionist, an orthomolecular psychiatrist, or a nutrition-oriented physician or chiropractor to have a supplement program tailor-made for your individual needs. Nowadays, most cities have holistic physicians who are well versed in the use of food supplements. To locate an orthomolecular psychiatrist, you might contact the Huxley Institute for Biosocial Research, 900 N. Federal Highway, Boca Raton, FL 33432, or the Academy for Orthomolecular Psychiatry, Nassau Mental Health Center, 1691 Northern Blvd., Manhasset, NY 11030.

If you elect to try vitamins and minerals on your own, the list on page 120, synthesized from all those recommended for sleep, should get you started.

L-TRYPTOPHAN

One of the most familiar folk remedies for insomnia is a glass of warm milk before bed. Not many experts take this bromide seriously, but strangely enough the milk does seem to help. Why? Is it soothing to the digestion, as some suggest? Is it the calcium? Or, as Freudians propose, is it subconsciously reminiscent of mother's milk?

People have long noted another soporific in daily use—a heavy meal. We tend to become drowsy after a big feast. Once it was thought this was caused by blood rushing from the head to the stomach, an explanation that turns out to be physiologically unsound.

The answer to both questions—the warm milk and the big meal—may have been discovered in the 1970s. Milk contains a high concentration of a certain essential amino acid; so do meats, fish, poultry, eggs, dairy products, nuts, soybeans, and other high-protein foods, the very things we usually gulp

PRO-SLEEP SUPPLEMENT CHART

Supplement	Effect on the Body	Recommended Daily Intake	Food Sources
Calcium	natural sedative important for nervous system	2 grams+	dairy products, bone meal
Magnesium	natural sedative aids in absorption of calcium	280 mgs	nuts, beets dates, prunes
Vitamin D	maintains nerve health, regulates calcium metabolism	2000 IU's	fish oil, eggs, milk, salmon, tuna
Vitamin E	maintains health of circulatory system, antioxident, reduces toxins in blood	400 IU's	green leafy vegetables, whole grains, wheat germ, vegetable oils
Vitamin B_6 (Pyridoxine)	natural sedative, regulates magnesium and tryptophan metabolism and protein metabolism	50 mgs	organ meats, whole grains, wheat germ, walnuts, peanuts, bananas, sunflower seeds, blackstrap molasses
Vitamin B_{12}	essential to health of nervous system, aids in carbohydrate metabolism, antistress effects	25 mgs	yeast, wheat germ, liver, milk, eggs and cheese
Niacinamide	maintains health of circulatory system, antistress effects, reduces tension	50 mgs 3× a day	yeast, organ meats, poultry, fish, wheat germ, nuts, soybeans
Inositol	controls cholesterol maintains health of brain tissue	1300 mgs	beef brain, beef heart, wheat germ, brown rice, brewer's yeast, molasses, nuts, citrus fruit

down in large quantities at a large meal. The amino acid is called *l-tryptophan,* and it became the subject of what many thought was a great breakthrough in the search for natural, safe methods for inducing sleep. Many felt that l-tryptophan was the long-sought-after sleeping pill without side effects.

After performing a number of l-tryptophan experiments at Boston State Hospital, Dr. Ernest Hartmann reported: "In our studies, we found that a dose of one gram of tryptophan will cut down the time it takes to fall asleep from 20 to 10 minutes. Its great advantage is that not only do you get to sleep sooner, but you do so without the distortions in sleep patterns that are produced by most sleeping pills."

Dr. Hartmann documented the effects of l-tryptophan on both rat and human subjects. All the human studies were comparisons of l-tryptophan in various doses with a placebo, under double-blind conditions where neither the patient nor the technicians and assistants knew its identity. L-tryptophan and the placebo were administered 20 minutes before bed-time, and records were kept of the usual physiological variables studied in the sleep labs. In addition to being measured for EEG and other physiological variables, the subjects—normal sleepers and insomniacs—filled out forms the next morning evaluating their sleep.

Dr. Hartmann summarized his results: "I believe these studies demonstrate that l-tryptophan is effective in reducing sleep latency [the amount of time it takes to fall asleep]. This is consistent with [the results obtained by other re-searchers]. . . . We have also shown that l-tryptophan defi-nitely increases subjective 'sleepiness' in normal subjects.

"There is general agreement that tryptophan reduces sleep latency, and usually reduces waking time; at low doses (1–5 grams) it does so without producing distortions of physiologi-cal sleep as measured by EEG recordings."

Why does l-tryptophan work? It is an essential amino acid that takes part in a number of metabolic processes, including the pathways that lead to proteins and polypeptides. It is directly linked to the production of serotonin, a neurotransmitter that apparently triggers the sleep mechanism. Explains Dr. Peter Hauri: "The tryptophan goes from the food into the blood and then to the brain, where it's converted into serotonin."

Administering l-tryptophan has been shown to increase serotonin levels, and that, in turn, might increase the receptivity to sleep. In studies with cats, an extreme reduction in serotonin levels has actually made it impossible for the animals to sleep for several days. Perhaps some cases of insomnia are caused or aggravated by insufficient serotonin levels, which might be rooted in l-tryptophan deficiencies in the diet or an inability to metabolize the substance properly.

Whatever the scientific explanation, l-tryptophan seems to help people get to sleep. It is not a drug that depresses the central nervous system. It is a naturally occurring substance; an l-tryptophan capsule would presumably fill a deficiency in the same way a vitamin or mineral tablet does, providing the body with an ingredient it normally takes in with food.

However, don't rush out to buy l-tryptophan. You might not find any, and if you do, you should check with your physician before taking it. In late 1989 l-tryptophan was linked to an outbreak in the southwest region of the United States of a rare blood disorder called eosinophilia. When it was learned that many of the 200 victims had been consuming l-tryptophan supplements, authorities removed the products from the market. As of this writing, there has been no final determination as to the cause of the outbreak or the possible role of the l-tryptophan supplements.

We spoke to many of the major sleep specialists who use l-tryptophan, and their responses were unanimous: if there is any link between the intake of l-tryptophan and eosinophilia, the cause is not likely to be the amino acid as such but rather some contaminant or foreign substance used in the manufacture of a specific product. (Some suspect that animal-grade l-tryptophan manufactured abroad was somehow packaged for humans.)

Many experts believe that the regular use of pure, pharmaceutical quality l-tryptophan manufactured in the United States should have no ill effects. In their minds, l-tryptophan remains, at this time, the preferred alternative to sleep medication. Bear in mind that until this recent scare, tens of thousands of people had used moderate doses of l-tryptophan to help them sleep and none had reported negative side effects.

L-tryptophan was researched and prescribed for over twenty years, and no side effects or toxicity were reported, even under high doses. According to a report on l-tryptophan from Great Britain, where the substance has been widely used in treating depression, doses of six to nine grams a day have been taken for a period of many months by several thousand patients with reports of very few side effects and no serious ones.

Before the controversy erupted, we had recommended l-tryptophan to a few insomniacs as an informal experiment, and we took it ourselves for several weeks. It seemed to work just as Dr. Hartmann described. Those who usually took a long time to go to sleep fell asleep a bit sooner; those who usually awakened prematurely either did not do so or fell back to sleep more quickly than usual. One person, who customarily awakened unrefreshed at dawn, took a gram of tryptophan at that time and fell back to sleep 15 minutes later. That, he claimed, was unprecedented.

Of course, we can't rule out psychological distortions in our informal experiment; a placebo effect is not unlikely. Everyone who tried it was excited by what they'd heard about l-tryptophan and wanted it very much to work. It is not inconceivable that all our subjects had good results simply because they wanted to and believed they would. That notwithstanding, those who took l-tryptophan in the recommended dosage did sleep better—as have subjects in rigorous laboratory studies, which control for psychological variables.

It should be noted that even before the eosinophilia outbreak, physicians who prescribed l-tryptophan counseled using it judiciously. Although it is apparently non–habit-forming, you would not want to use it as a crutch or run the risk of becoming psychologically dependent on it or *any* substance. Think of it as a supplement that can be discontinued after it redresses an amino acid deficiency, not as a sleeping pill to be used indefinitely.

If returned to the shelves, l-tryptophan would be available in well-stocked health-food stores and pharmacies. Two 500 mg capsules provide the 1 gram that Dr. Hartmann recommends taking 20 minutes before bed. In addition, you might want to eat foods that contain substantial amounts of l-tryptophan.

However, although l-tryptophan is abundant in high-protein foods, some experts feel high-protein meals are not the best way to boost l-tryptophan levels in the brain. They theorize that the other amino acids in high-protein foods compete with l-tryptophan for the carrier molecules that transport amino acids to the brain. In this view, high-carbohydrate meals are more likely to stimulate production of serotonin because the insulin such meals release transports competing amino acids into body tissue, thereby freeing l-tryptophan for uptake to the brain.

This hypothesis was tested by Dr. Hartmann and MIT's Richard Wurtman, who gave volunteers either high-protein or high-carbohydrate meals. Two hours later, the carbohydrate eaters were significantly more sleepy than those who ate protein. Whether this would always be the case, whether one group slept *better* than the other, whether changing the *form* of carbohydrate and protein eaten would make a difference—these and other questions remain to be answered. More research is needed before we know the best way to raise l-tryptophan levels. In the meantime, here is a rundown of the amounts of l-tryptophan in common foods.

FOODS RICH IN L-TRYPTOPHAN

Food	Portion	Amount of L-tryptophan (mg)
Dairy Products		
American cheese	1 oz.	98
Cheddar cheese	1 oz.	98
Parmesan cheese	1 oz.	140
Swiss cheese	1 oz.	100
Cottage cheese	1 cup	336
Sour cream	1 cup	94
Whole milk	½ pint	119
Nonfat, fortified milk	½ pint	137
Egg	large	112
Meats and Fish		
Hamburger	¼ lb.	255
Chicken (fryer)	1⅓ oz.	115
Pork chop	1 oz.	96
Pot roast	½ lb.	319
Sirloin steak	½ lb.	373
T-bone steak	½ lb.	281
Lamb chop	½ lb.	379
Veal cutlet	3½ oz.	435
Halibut	1 fish	208
Tuna (canned)	¾ cup	914
Nuts		
Cashews	6–8	64
Peanuts (roasted)	20	67
Peanut butter	1 oz.	109
Other:		
Oatmeal, dry	1 cup	146
Green peas	½ cup	34
Spinach	½ cup	47
Rice (white)	1 cup	157
Pasta	½ cup	60
Lima beans	⅝ cup	68

We conclude with our Basic Pro-Sleep Eating Plan:

Be moderate. Overeating makes excessive demands on the body. Insomniacs should be especially conservative in the evening, as overeating will obstruct sleep. Your body can't rest if it is working overtime to digest a big meal.

Cut down on fatty foods and greasy, hard-to-digest dishes.

Eat only when you are hungry. Trust your body, not the clock.

Chew thoroughly and eat slowly. Digestion begins in the mouth.

Try not to eat when you are emotionally upset or over-tired.

Avoid chemical preservatives and additives as much as possible. Studies with hyperactive children have shown improvement, in most cases, as soon as these were eliminated from their diets.

Avoid, or cut down on, sugar and white flour.

CHAPTER 7

Physicians for the Soul: Your Emotions and Your Sleep

The greatest mistake in the treatment of diseases is that there are physicians for the body and physicians for the soul, although the two cannot be separated.

PLATO

It has been over 2,000 years since Plato made his sage observation, yet we still act as though our minds and bodies can somehow be treated independently of each other. As we stated earlier, some see insomnia as a problem of the body; others see it as a problem of the mind. Experts have come to recognize the holistic nature of insomnia, but when treating it they tend to put their attention on one side or the other. Most specialists have neither the skill nor the time to gain expertise in more than one discipline. But for an insomniac, it's important to understand how our attitudes, moods, values, perceptions, and methods of handling problems influence our sleep.

In some cases, sleeplessness is a sign of a serious mental disorder. Both schizophrenics and manic-depressive psychotics tend to manifest sleep difficulties along with the more tragic symptoms of those diseases, but for the most part insomnia is associated with the classic neurotic symptoms with which most of us are familiar. Through tests and interviews it has been determined that insomniacs, as a group, are anxious, introverted, and prone to psychosomatic illness. According to Dr. Quentin Regestein, "Many chronic insomniac patients are described as tense, complaining, histrionic individuals, who are oversensitive to minor discomforts and unable to relax easily."

In discussing the causes of insomnia with psychiatrists and psychologists, we found that there is a wide range of theories to account for the problem. They range from the superanalytical—"Some neurotics feel so weak and vulnerable that they are afraid they will die during sleep" (maybe Mark Twain wasn't kidding when he advised, "Don't go to bed, because so many people die there")—to the superbehaviorist— "Sleeplessness is a learned, or conditioned, response to a certain set of stimuli." The recommended treatments are equally diverse.

Most experts feel that the two principal types of insomnia are correlated with the two principal categories of emotional problems: difficulty falling asleep is linked to anxiety; trouble staying asleep is associated with depression. Although that categorization strikes us as somewhat facile (in our experience, there are many exceptions to the rule), it is so widely accepted by sleep specialists that there must be some empirical basis for it. In any event, depression and anxiety are certainly among the leading contenders for causes of insomnia.

DEALING WITH DEPRESSION

Of all emotional problems, depression is the one most commonly associated with insomnia. Sadness seems to seep into sleep in an insidious manner, and depression is sadness that has gone beyond what is justified by actual events. Unlike anger and rage, which manifest physically in ways that obviously work against sleep, depression just keeps yanking at the bedcovers for no apparent reason, and it seems to run in a vicious cycle—depression wakes you up, the fact that you can't sleep makes you feel even more depressed and helpless, and on it goes.

The sleep clinic at New York's Montefiore Hospital defines depression this way: "An emotional illness characterized by feelings of sadness, hopelessness, worthlessness, and guilt. It may be mild, resulting from neurosis or a crisis in the patient's life. Neurotic depression is believed to be a 'learned' psychopathology caused by longstanding inappropriate mechanisms of integrating experiences into emotional life. Other forms of depression are severe, and are apparently innate, biochemically and/or genetically determined illnesses."

Studies indicate that depressed persons have less than the normal amount of Stages III and IV of sleep. They also have shorter sleep times and more frequent awakenings. Early morning awakenings are associated with *endogenous depression,* a more or less self-inflicted, chronic state of sadness, not precipitated by any particular outside circumstance.

How can one deal with depression? Severe and prolonged cases are often treated with antidepressant drugs, progress on which has advanced to the point where many of the earlier side effects have been eliminated. Drug treatment, of course, must be prescribed and monitored by a psychiatrist. Despite the advances in antidepressants, however, dependency on drugs is still anathema for many psychiatrists, so they tend to combine drug therapy with other procedures and wean the patient off the medicine as quickly as possible. Others, of course, use the many varieties of talk therapy, ranging from classical Freudian analysis to the newer "growth therapies" that have spun off from human potential research. Cognitive therapy has earned high marks in recent years, and certain behavioral approaches have been found effective. Still other experts use orthomolecular treatments, relying on mega-vitamins and amino acids to correct physiological imbalances that may affect the brain.

If you are looking for a therapist, your local college or university's psychology department is a good referral source, as is your physician. In most large population areas, state or local mental-health associations or a branch of the American Psychiatric Association can provide a list of qualified therapists. Reference books can aid your search: *The Directory of Approved Counseling Agencies* gives a complete list of accredited places from which you can obtain therapy; *The Complete Guide to Therapy: From Psychoanalysis to Behavior Modification* by Dr. Joel Kovel summarizes the various options available.

For the average insomniac, the problem is not likely to be pathological depression but the everyday sadness that afflicts each of us at one time or another. Everyone has his or her own ways of dealing with the clouds that cast shadows on our psyches. A fun movie, a concert, a walk in the woods, a visit with cheerful friends or relatives, or some time with a favorite hobby are all activities that can warm the heart, inspire the imagination, and lighten the mind, especially in the evening prior to bedtime. Also, nothing is as uplifting as simple beauty. Both nature and art rejuvenate the soul. They reveal our roots in the fabric of creation, remind us that life is more than a series of problems, and demonstrate that love, joy, and happiness are within everyone's grasp.

With respect to evening entertainment, it might be wise to select humorous fare rather than an unsettling thriller or a ponderous, intense drama that might remind you of your troubles and keep you up thinking. In the best-selling *Anatomy of an Illness*, Norman Cousins wrote about the time he was hospitalized for an apparently terminal illness, during which he slept horribly. He had a film projector installed in his room and proceeded to watch Marx Brothers' movies and old "Candid Camera" episodes. The humor not only provided him with hours of pain-free sleep, but it actually altered the course of his disease.

Many people derive great solace and inspiration from their religious traditions. A visit to your church or temple, or a talk with your minister, rabbi, or priest might help renew your faith in both yourself and the universe. Persons who are not religiously inclined often get a similar spiritual boost from contemplating the discoveries of science. Standing on a beach at night, looking up at the distant galaxies, and meditating on the immensity of the universe and our place in it is often a good way to put the petty cares of the day in their proper perspective. Awe, wonder, and reverence are such powerfully positive emotions that they can often overshadow the most stubborn blues.

We mention these time-tested palliatives even though they might seem self-evident because they are often overlooked just when they are needed most. Persons ridden with cares and woes, which are often taken out of perspective and exaggerated, sometimes feel that they cannot afford the time or energy to "indulge" in diversions. They feel they need to weigh their problems at all times, and when they are not doing so they feel guilty of escaping or turning away. If that sounds familiar, you need to tell yourself to stop being obsessed with the negative, at least for the course of a night's sleep.

This is not to advocate escapism. Indeed, most psychologists agree that for an insomniac understanding your feelings is vital, and confronting your problems—inner and outer—is necessary for any permanent improvement. Furthermore, ignoring your feelings can, in the long run, be more damaging than honest confrontation; they will find an outlet eventually, often with terribly inappropriate timing. Meanwhile, your repressed emotions can eat away at you subconsciously and keep you awake at night.

However, you needn't deal with them by obsessing at

bedtime. "Our sleep," wrote the great psychotherapist Alfred Adler, "can be undisturbed only if we are free from tension and sure of the solution of our problem."

If your depression is chronic, you are well-advised to see a counselor or psychiatrist. For assistance, advice, and nationwide referrals, you might also contact the Foundation for Depression and Manic Depression in New York. Their phone number is (212) 772-3400. Here are some general points from mental-health experts on dealing with everyday depression:

Evaluate yourself candidly, admitting your weaknesses and acknowledging your strengths. Then set out to decrease the former, strengthen the latter, and accept what you can't change.

Learn to find satisfaction in doing the things that suit you best rather than longing for the impossible.

Look forward to where you want to go and what you want yourself to be—don't dwell on past failures. Assess your mistakes, learn from them, and move on.

Take responsibility for both your present condition and your future. Remember that your life is yours to make of it what you will. You are not a helpless pawn in the hands of fate, even if it seems that way.

Whenever you begin mentally to berate yourself for your inadequacies, just stop. Exert your will. Negative thoughts never do any good and almost always defeat you.

If you are beset by serious problems, resolve to face up to them. Get help. Simply deciding on an initial course of action might ease your mind enough to open the doors to slumber.

ATTACKING ANXIETY

Anxiety, with its attendant fear and worry, is perhaps the most pernicious of the sleep-robbing emotions. If you are lying awake unable to fall asleep, chances are that your thoughts are worries and fears. In all likelihood a good percentage of the things you are worrying about are either relatively trivial or matters about which you can do nothing.

Some habitual worrying can be cleared away by the right diet, relaxation, exercise, or other physical treatments. Physiological imbalances and general tension can color our moods, causing us to evaluate negatively everything we perceive. But for many people such cures are insufficient—only expert therapy or strong conscious effort will change the habits of their minds.

To the extent that worry is a learned response that can be unlearned, you can attack the habit with mental energy. For example, you might do well to cultivate what Bertrand Russell called "the habit of thinking of things at the right time." Avoid idle speculation about the future, Russell implored, and don't let yourself worry uselessly about the inevitable, or about things over which you have no control. To do otherwise is only a waste of time, and it will gnaw away at your sanity and your sleep.

With respect to the intractable problems that keep us awake worrying, Russell says, "The wise man thinks about his troubles only when there is some purpose in doing so; at other times he thinks about other things, or, if at night, about nothing at all." Contemplate a problem only when it is relevant, practical, and all the information you need is available. Above all, don't try to solve your problems while lying in bed hoping to fall asleep. When you are tired, your ability to think rationally and evaluate the situation clearly is impaired, so it's hardly the most opportune moment to make decisions. The facts will probably not change overnight, so tell yourself that the most practical approach is to get some sleep and deal with it in the morning when your mind is clear and your body refreshed, and you will be able to act on your decisions.

Some psychologists conjecture that insomniacs often avoid sleep because of a sense of guilt—they feel that by sleeping they are turning their backs on their problems. They might even fear that if they stop thinking about their miseries the solution will somehow evade them. This is nonsense. The mind needs rest so that it can return to the business at hand refreshed. And return it will, if the problems are real (and if they are not, good riddance). Indeed, falling asleep may be the most practical way to find a solution. Many great discoveries slipped into the discoverer's mind during dreams or immediately on awakening; the subconscious often works at synthesizing knowledge while the conscious mind sleeps.

Jane Turner, a schoolteacher, claims she cured her insomnia by learning how to control her anxiety. She systematically attacked her worries. "I got into the habit of sitting down and asking myself if the situation really warrants all that much concern. Nine times out of 10, it does not. Often, the whole thing seems truly ridiculous when examined in an objective light."

Turner said that sometimes she required a friend's ear to supplement her own: "I would find an intelligent, sincere, and optimistic person—the more cheerful the better. Somehow, articulating my fears and hearing them as if from someone else's point of view brought out how very ludicrous some of my worries were."

Often anxiety is vague and free-floating, a sort of generalized apprehension, fear, or sense of frustration. But in most cases the mind needs something concrete to which to attach such feelings. You can't just worry—you have to worry *about* something. You can't just be afraid—you have to be afraid *of* something. So, you connect the free-floating emotion to something or someone in your life at that time, focus on it, and often become obsessed. Usually, it is not worth the energy, for the worry actually has no basis in reality.

"When misfortune threatens," says Bertrand Russell, "consider seriously and deliberately what is the very worst that could possibly happen. Having looked this possible misfortune in the face, give yourself sound reasons for thinking that after all it would be no such very terrible disaster."

Richard Wynn, a New York City accountant, helped his insomnia by discovering the difference between concern and worry. It's a useful distinction indeed. "I never really understood the difference between concern and worry," he said. "Finally, it occurred to me that worrying never helps you solve a problem. If anything, it gets in the way of intelligent solutions. To worry is to admit defeat before the battle. I learned instead to be concerned, in a healthy way, about things that were important."

Instead of anticipating disaster, think back to a time when you made it through a tough situation and take inspiration from that. Try not to think of such troublesome situations as problems but as challenges to your strength and opportunities for growth. "What doesn't kill me makes me stronger," Friedrich Nietzsche wrote.

Worry is usually an outgrowth of fear, and many of us are chronically, irrationally afraid. We are afraid of poverty, death, illness, failure, loss of love, and countless other disasters. The real tragedy is that, with the exception of death, all these fearsome events are usually in our control. We act as though they are not, but in fact we mostly determine our own losses and gains. Being afraid is not only a waste of time, it's tantamount to admitting that we do not trust ourselves.

It is far more useful to devote your energy to running your life in such a way as to avert or prevent the dangers before they come. If you do in fact lack confidence, your only solution is to build yourself into the kind of person in whom you will have confidence. If you do that, you will not lose sleep worrying. Great people, those who assume great responsibilities, often sleep as soundly as babes. Certainly they have as much to worry about as the rest of us, if not more, but no amount of pressure can disturb their sleep. The difference is they are not afraid. They know they can handle almost anything that comes their way. "I would no sooner lose to insomnia," said a football coach who was known to sleep on buses and in the locker room, "than I would to a rival football team."

Franklin D. Roosevelt's famous words are never more true than when your head hits the pillow: "We have nothing to fear but fear itself."

Try to give your mind more desirable, positive thoughts to ponder. When you find yourself overwhelmed by anxiety, you can choose instead to look at the brighter side. Many of us have caught the spirit of pessimism that has gripped the modern age. We have come to accept disappointment and frustration as inevitable. Many authorities, however, believe the act of *thinking* that tragedy is inevitable is what makes it so. Why not turn it around? Perhaps by thinking that tragedy is unnecessary and that happiness is your birthright, you can make happiness inevitable. If you work at it, positive emotions can become a habitual way of thinking. If positivity doesn't bring you true happiness, it might at least bring you a good night's sleep.

None of this is meant to suggest that you develop a blasé attitude or an ostrichlike disregard for problems. Denial will do about as much to promote sound sleep as a cup of black coffee. However, if you look at an anxiety-causing situation with true objectivity you are compelled to look at the positive side as well as the negative. The positive perspective is always there if you look hard enough and are prepared to lose the strange security that many people seem to find in believing that the cards are stacked against them. The key—and it is a delicate one—is to balance positivity with realism.

"Kill the habit of worry, in all its forms," advises Napoleon Hill, author of *Think and Grow Rich*, "by reaching a general, blanket decision that nothing which life has to offer is worth the price of worry. With this decision will come poise, peace of mind, and calmness of thought which will bring happiness." And, we must add, sound sleep! But don't try to drive negative thoughts from your mind forcibly. Be gentle and patient—old habits are not broken easily.

Here is a practical suggestion from psychiatrist Harold Bloomfield: "If you are troubled by fears write them *all* down until you are completely exhausted. Then destroy them all that night by burning them or tearing them up. Then go to sleep. In the morning, you'll have a fresh perspective. Repeat this nightly for as long as it takes for the fears to go away."

HELP FROM BOOKS

There is no substitute for competent professional help when depression or anxiety chronically rob you of sleep, but you can find expert advice from some highly qualified authors of books. Here are some of the best (* indicates books the authors have found particularly valuable):

*The Conquest of Happiness, by Bertrand Russell. New York: Liveright, 1958.

Depression and Its Treatment, by John Greist. Washington, D.C.: American Psychiatric Press, 1984.

Depression Hits Every Family, by Grace Ketterman, M.D. Nashville: Thomas Nelson, 1988.

Fighting Fear, by Melvin Neumann, M.D. New York: Macmillan, 1985.

Getting Undepressed, by Gary Emery, Ph.D. New York: Simon and Schuster, 1981.

The Good News about Panic, Anxiety and Phobias, by Mark Gold, M.D. New York: Villard Books, 1989.

Managing Your Anxiety, by Christopher J. McCullough, Ph.D. Los Angeles: Jeremy P. Tarcher, 1985.

*Mastering the Problems of Living, by Haridas Chaudhuri. New York: Citadel Press, 1960.

No More Fears, by Douglas Hunt, M.D. New York: Warner Books, 1988.

*You Are Not the Target, by Laura Huxley. Los Angeles: Jeremy P. Tarcher, 1986.

*The Way Up From Down, by Priscilla Slagle, M.D. New York: Random House, 1987.

DON'T WORRY, BE SLEEPY

One form of anxiety is what every insomniac worries about and is the one fear that kills more sleep than any other. It is also the one worry that least deserves to be a worry: the fear that you won't be able to sleep.

There are three reasons not to lose sleep over losing sleep. One, it does no good—the worrying itself will keep you awake as surely as any other cause of insomnia. Two, even if you *do* get a bad night's sleep, the actual harm done will be easily reversible, not permanent. Three, you may not have insomnia in the first place.

Herbert Spencer, the nineteenth-century philosopher, once lived in a boardinghouse, where he would aggravate his fellow tenants with constant complaints about his insomnia. He was so obsessed with his problem that he took opium and used earplugs in hope of curing it. One night he shared his room with a professor friend of his. In the morning, Spencer declared, as usual, that he hadn't slept a wink all night. "Neither did I," replied the professor. "Your snoring kept me awake."

Spencer was not the first person to suffer from what is called *pseudoinsomnia* and he wasn't the last. Every sleep expert has at least one good story on the subject. Says Dr. Richard J. Wyatt of the National Institute of Mental Health: "All physicians are aware of subjective complaints of patients who report that they haven't slept for days or months. When these same patients are hospitalized and are under the scrutiny of a nursing staff checking for sleep throughout the night, it is invariably reported that the patient is in fact sleeping . . . and for long periods."

Dr. William C. Dement, pioneer sleep researcher at Stanford University, says that "although *every* insomniac came to our clinic as his 'last hope' in getting some respite from the tortures of sleeplessness, the severity of their complaint had *absolutely no relation* to the amount they slept in the laboratory."

Dement and his colleagues related this unusual story in *Psychology Today*: "A real estate broker, Barry G., . . . had been forced into early retirement, he told us, by loss of sleep at night and a consequent fatigue during the day. He reported that each evening he lay awake an hour or more, then woke up uneasily several times in the night and could never sleep beyond 5 o'clock in the morning. He averaged less than five hours a night, he said, and his wife told us that he was obsessed with the need to get 'his proper sleep.' He got no relief from pills or psychiatry. When we asked him to keep a diary and to record his daytime feeling of sleepiness every 15 minutes, he confirmed his complaints in great detail.

"But when he came to the clinic for two all-night sleep recordings, his body told a very different story. He was a normal sleeper. He actually fell asleep in less than 10 minutes and was awake for only 20 minutes all night. He spent 7 hours and 13 minutes in normal sleep."

Often, a person who confronts the fact of his pseudoinsomnia by seeing the evidence in a sleep clinic needs nothing more. The patient described above sent the Stanford clinic this letter three months after he was told that he slept normally:

"Now that I know that I get a normal amount of sleep I don't fret and worry about sleeping. I seem to awaken less frequently during the night. It is a relief not to use sleeping tablets any more, as they made me dopey and depressed. I find that nowadays I am not particularly depressed."

That patient discovered what many other insomniacs have: worrying over sleep loss is a more certain way to lose sleep than having a pneumatic drill pound outside your bedroom window. Psychologists have coined a word for it— *agrypniaphobia,* a somewhat unpronounceable word that simply means "fear of insomnia."

Why do people think they don't sleep when they actually do? One reason might be a form of hypochondria. Some people have a need to have something wrong with them. Why not insomnia? Another reason might be exceptionally light sleep. So-called "poor sleepers" have been found statistically to underestimate the actual time spent sleeping far more than "good sleepers."

Gay Gaer Luce, coauthor of *Insomnia,* suggests that "the

sleeper remembers only the last stage of sleep, when he is close to awakening. Thus, although the lab monitors that he slept 6 hours, he thinks he slept only 20 minutes. Or it may be that all of the person's sleeping is spent in a very light stage of sleep."

Another theory is that the person may sleep normally but *dream* he is awake. A student at Dartmouth once went to Peter Hauri's sleep lab complaining that he could not sleep. In the clinic, it was determined that he slept a full eight hours. Yet he was exhausted in the morning. Analysis revealed that he had been dreaming he was not asleep.

Whatever the reason, you may in fact be getting a lot more sleep than you think you are. People who toss and turn a great deal are likely to turn minutes into hours in their imaginations. Experts agree that even long periods of nighttime wakefulness are punctuated by brief periods of genuine sleep.

Another reason you may be misconceiving your problem is that you may simply need less sleep than you think you do. We have all grown up with the notion that everyone must sleep eight hours a night. Not so. There is no rule as to the proper length of time that any one of us should sleep. According to a 1962 survey, 61 percent sleep the customary eight hours, 23 percent sleep less than eight (with 8 percent sleeping less than five hours), and 15 percent sleep at least nine hours.

Dr. Hauri tells of a 70-year-old woman "whose husband sent her to the clinic because he thought she had a sleep disorder: she only slept four hours a night. She told me that she hadn't ever slept much more than four hours a night in her whole life—she thought it was peculiar too. Well, we tested her in the laboratory, and there was nothing at all wrong. What she did have was a remarkably efficient sleep. She went very quickly into deep delta slumber, the Stage III and IV phases. And then, after about an hour and a half of that, up she came. She went directly into a little REM dream period. After that, back down she went, came out once more, and then it was all over. And if she didn't have more than a tiny bit of the Stage I or Stage II intermediate stuff, it was because she didn't actually need more than the four hours of sleep. She was as sound as a bell."

How much sleep do you need? Only you know. Some people have been known to do with very little, among them Napoleon, Edison, Churchill, Gladstone, and Goethe. The great architect and philosopher R. Buckminster Fuller slept only four hours a day—in half-hour naps every three hours around the clock. He thrived on that schedule until he had to give it up because he was so out of tune with the rest of us. Other celebrities who don't spend much time in bed include consumer advocate Ralph Nader, who rose to fame on four-and-a-half hours of sleep (he now needs five or six), and super-model Jerry Hall, who says she needs only five hours sleep since she increased the amount of vegetables in her diet.

There are unverified claims of exceptional people, such as some yogis in India who allegedly need hardly any sleep at all, but the record for verified short sleep belongs to two Australian men, aged 30 and 54, who needed less than three hours a night. Then there is the case of Valentine Medina, a 75-year-old Spaniard who farmed by day and patrolled his village by night. According to *The Guinness Book of World Records*, Medina claimed to have lost all desire to sleep in 1904 and not to have slept after that. Said Señor Medina, "I've taken sleeping pills until I rattle, but it does no good."

Guinness also records the longest period of voluntary sleep deprivation: 282 hours and 55 minutes (over 11 days), a record held by Bertha Van Der Merwe, a South African house-wife, aged 52 at the time. Closer to home, an American high-school student named Randy Gardner once stayed awake, with a little help from his friends, for 264 hours and 12 minutes. Randy did this to break the record of Peter Tripp, the New York disc jockey whose 200-hour publicity "wakathon" we mentioned earlier.

On the flip side of the pillow are inveterate sleepers such

as comedian-composer Steve Allen. In addition to his regular TV appearances, Allen has written numerous books and thousands of songs, yet he sleeps 11 hours a night. To make up for lost time he keeps a pencil and pad at his bedside. His biggest hit, "This Could Be the Start of Something Big," reportedly came to him in a dream.

There are several lessons in these examples, each of which should help you to cut down on the amount of worrying you do over what may or may not be insomnia. First, as we've mentioned, all the studies on sleep deprivation have shown that people recover astoundingly well, even from severe sleep loss. "One thing we have learned," reports British psychologist, R. T. Wilkinson, "is that if people want to maintain normal performance, it's surprising how well they can." He was referring to the insomniac's ability to perform as expected following a bout with sleeplessness.

Researchers have found a definite correlation between physical and emotional strength and a person's ability to recover from sleep loss. Highly motivated, confident, healthy people perform better following an interrupted night's sleep than do chronic complainers, worriers, and the insecure. The thing to remember is, if you want to function well you can still do so despite having lost some sleep. Knowing that insomnia need not ruin your life, or even your day, should help you eliminate the anxiety that will, by creating a vicious worry-go-round, keep you awake again the next night.

Another lesson to glean from this discussion is not to force your sleep pattern into some preconceived notion of how long you ought to sleep. Determine your own natural sleep requirement and your most efficient pattern, and use that as your sole yardstick. Your inner rhythms might be different from the pattern dictated by social customs. Most of us respect individuality enough to accept the fact that some people eat less or more than others. We tolerate the fact that different people have different needs with respect to money, exercise, sex, and everything else. Why not the same for sleep?

Many people think they are insomniacs because they can't get to sleep "on time." Richard Campbell, a 56-year-old lawyer, thought for years that he had insomnia. He would get to bed at 11 and proceed to toss fitfully for two to three hours. In the morning he would struggle out of bed with the alarm clock reverberating in his cloudy head and trudge off to the office. Eventually, a passing remark from a friend saved his life: "Why don't you just stay up?"

Campbell had never heard such a sensible remark. He started to go to sleep when he felt tired, not when the clock told him to. He fell asleep within minutes every night. Of course, he wanted to sleep later as well, so he rearranged his schedule, never making appointments before 10 A.M. unless absolutely necessary. In all, he made much better use of his 24-hour day.

The reverse is also common. Betty Nichols, a Boston schoolteacher, used to awaken at dawn, never fully refreshed. She would lie in bed until forced out by the need to make breakfast for her children, then proceed exhausted to school. It turned out that Ms. Nichols was a dedicated Johnny Carson fan and forced herself to stay awake to see his show. Then one week Carson was on vacation and his replacement did not appeal to Nichols at all. She took the opportunity to go to bed earlier. She woke up at dawn, as usual, but now she felt refreshed.

Betty Nichols's internal clock was geared to an early-to-bed, early-to-rise routine, but she had been fighting it. Once she adapted to her natural rhythm she no longer sleepwalked through the day and she made good use of the hour just before the rest of her family awakened—she watched a tape of the previous night's "Johnny Carson Show."

Other people who should not worry about insomnia include *polyphasic* sleepers. Some of us would be better off sleeping in separate stages than in one long session. If you awaken in the night and feel alert and unable to get back to sleep, and if you find that you are tired during the day, you might fall into this category. Try getting out of bed and doing something constructive when you can't fall back to sleep. If doing this and going back to sleep later on—or napping during the day—feels right, you might consider institutionalizing a two-phase sleep pattern.

Dr. Roger Williams, a biochemist at the University of Texas, describes his experience of polyphasic sleep in his book *You Are Extraordinary:* "I do not regard my condition as a disease; if it is, it is an attractive one for me. My mind is clearest during this hour or so and I reserve this time to do my best thinking. I go to bed with problems unsolved, but when I get up in the morning after having had this quiet hour in the night, the best solution I can devise inevitably comes to me."

One very important fact to bear in mind is that sleep needs tend to diminish with age. "Nothing changes so measurably between the ages of 20 and 50 as sleep," says Dr. Irwin Feinberg of the Fort Miley Veterans Administration Hospital in San Francisco. "Deep sleep is reduced by 60 percent. The number of arousals in the night doubles. People over 70 spend more time in bed, but less time asleep. Their sleep is constantly fragmented, disturbed by awakenings."

Dr. Feinberg's statement is echoed by every sleep expert. A publication from Montefiore describes this pattern: "Sleep efficiency decreases after 30 years in men and 50 years in women, then decreases more steeply in both sexes after the mid-50s. The number of awakenings per night increases gradually until 40 years in men and 70 years in women, then increases more steeply after those ages."

Just knowing these facts and allowing themselves the privilege of napping as often as they need has kept many older persons away from sleeping pills. Others are not so fortunate. "People who get older need less sleep," says University of Cincinnati psychiatrist Milton Kramer, "but because they've been raised on the myth of 'a normal eight hours sleep,' they're likely to be the first customers for all those sleeping pills on the market that end up doing more harm than good."

Another thing to be aware of is that waking in the night is relatively normal, especially as we age. According to Dr. Hauri, adults generally awaken three to five times during a healthy night's sleep. Most people return to sleep instantly and do not remember having awakened. It is those who do remember that often become alarmed unnecessarily. If you find yourself aroused at night, the only important questions to ask are, Does it take excessively long to fall back to sleep? and Are you tired during the day?

DON'T WORRY, BE CONCERNED

In determining whether, in fact, your sleep problems are really worthy of concern and not something easily adjusted to with proper understanding or a new schedule, keep in mind that your sleep needs may vary with circumstances. For example, you might need more sleep during periods of crisis or change, or when you are under emotional stress. Many women often need more sleep during pregnancy or their menstrual period; other women might experience temporary insomnia at those times. Changes in your work schedule or social life, a new diet or unusual meals, getting more exercise or less—these are all examples of conditions that might throw your sleep temporarily out of whack and trick you into thinking you have insomnia.

Knowing the facts might eliminate you from the category of insomniacs. If you are still unsure whether your problem is really a problem, there are certain key factors you should consider before deciding whether the condition warrants action:

• How dramatically has your sleep changed?
• How long have the disturbances lasted?
• How severe are the attendant signs of emotional instability and loss of efficiency?

If the change in your sleep pattern has been dramatic and persistent, if lethargy, irritability, poor coordination, lapses of attention, chronic fatigue, and other side effects are present, then you have good reason to be concerned.

But you still have no reason to worry. Even if your insomnia is genuine, it can be overcome. You need nothing more than, well, a good night's sleep. That's probably easier to obtain than you think. If none of the natural remedies presented here does the trick, then seek professional help. The fact is, your body simply will not tolerate sleeplessness for too long, just as it will not tolerate hunger.

Until you find the answer to your particular condition, here is a thought to comfort you and keep you from bemoaning your sleeplessness too much: It could be worse. When F. Scott Fitzgerald wrote, "The worst thing in the world is to try to sleep and not to," he may have failed to consider the opposite situation: the person who wants to be awake but sleeps instead.

Studies have shown that people with *hypersomnia* suffer the same kinds of difficulties as insomniacs. But these unfortunate people don't even get to enjoy being awake. At least insomniacs have time to read!

It is wise not to worry about your loss of sleep and even wiser not to worry about *getting* to sleep. Worrying about not falling asleep is likely to be self-fulfilling.

Still, if all our reasons fail to prevent you from worrying about sleep, pin up this terse reminder from sleep expert Dr. Nathaniel Kleitman: "No one ever died of insomnia."

CHAPTER 8

How to Court Sleep at Bedtime

Sleep is the most moronic fraternity in the world, with the heaviest dues and the crudest rituals.

VLADIMIR NABOKOV

*I*t may be moronic, but sleep is one fraternity to which we would all like a lifetime membership. So far, most of our discussion has centered on how to overcome the physical and psychological reasons why so many of us have been excluded from the club. Our suggestions have dealt mainly with things to do during the day—ways to improve your mental and physical health, and by extension your sleep. But there are also helpful ways to encourage the sandman at night.

Some of those crude rituals to which Nabokov referred can be pretty bizarre. Sleep researcher Gay Gaer Luce describes a man who paints his face white and goes to sleep in a coffin. "He has a thing about death," says Ms. Luce, "and the only way he can resolve it is to actively play dead." Others are less weird but still humorously idiosyncratic. Van Gogh insisted he could sleep only on a pillow made of hops, a ritual that has a long history in folklore. Abraham Lincoln always took a long midnight walk. Catherine the Great would not go to sleep until her servant brushed her hair 100 times.

We all have our own rituals, and even the simple ones are indispensable; we don't feel quite right about going to bed without them. If you don't believe you are dependent on pre-bed rituals, try sleeping in a strange place where you can't follow your customary routine. Try going to bed without brushing your teeth, watching the late news, reading, locking the door, wearing pajamas, or getting a glass of whatever it is you are accustomed to drinking.

If you do not have an identifiable routine or ritual, that may be part of your problem. Maybe you need to find one that works for you and make it a habit. Conversely, perhaps your established ritual is actually interfering with your sleep. There is no universal formula, of course, but there are certain features that good rituals should have. In this chapter, we will discuss the proper way to approach your evening activities and manage your environment so as to induce sleep.

Actually, the word *induce* might not be quite appropriate. "The idea of 'inducing sleep' is absurd," wrote Arnold Bennett. "Sleep ought not to have to be enticed like a frightened fawn. It should pounce on you like a tiger."

True enough, but why not do all we can to bait the trap?

WINDING DOWN

You should start preparing for bed long before your actual bedtime. Dr. Dean Foster, consultant to the Sleep Research Foundation, once wrote: "Going to sleep is like stopping a car at an intersection. A driver who sees a traffic light change a block away is better off slowing down gradually and coasting to a stop, rather than coming to a sudden brake-slamming halt. Taper off your day's activities before getting ready for bed."

In our chapter on stress, we reminded you to try to leave your work at the office. Start winding down when you get home. That is a good time to exercise, meditate, take a walk with your spouse, play with your children, catch up on some reading, or whatever. If you have troubled sleep, it is *not* the time to worry about the next day at work or to review all your problems. If your work is so aggravating that you consistently can't get it off your mind, you should seriously consider whether or not it's worth it.

If you must bring paperwork home with you, get it done early in the evening, or stop at least an hour before bedtime. Your late-night reading should be unrelated to work and not something that requires concentrated effort. If you read fiction, it should be entertaining—but save the gripping suspense or horror for the weekends. It might also be wise to choose late-night reading with short chapters or sections so you can read to a logical stopping point and go to sleep with no loose ends. A collection of short stories might be a good idea.

Psychoanalyst Edward Bauer, who used to have trouble falling asleep, claims to have solved his problem by switching reading matter. "I used to read the case histories of my next day's patients before bed," he says, "but I got so worked up planning how to deal with these troubled people that I couldn't fall asleep. Finally, I took to reading the histories on the train home. I still have to read before bed, but now I read detective stories—short ones. I've been through all of Sherlock Holmes and I sleep like a baby."

Another person whose reading habits changed his sleep was John Wagner, a publicist at a publishing house. "I like to read in bed," says Wagner, "but I used to read the books of authors we were working with. It got me thinking too much about publicity campaigns." A philosophical man, Wagner switched to his favorite theologian, Thomas Merton, and always ends his evening with a selection from one of Merton's books. "I fall asleep soothed and inspired by a great man's words," he says.

Spiritual works are often favored by people who read themselves to sleep. It is more than superstition and more than the fervor of the Gideon Society that makes the Bible a common fixture on hotel end tables. For spiritual persons nothing is more soothing or more elevating than inspirational writings. Poetry is also a good bet, especially lyrical works, and you can't miss with Shakespeare if you stick to the comedies and avoid getting wired by *Othello* or *Macbeth*.

What about other nighttime entertainment? The same rules apply. If you are a movie fan, a theater buff, or a TV viewer, try to keep the fare light as you approach sleeptime. If you are drawn to an action thriller or a heavy drama, go to the movies early and give yourself time to wind down afterward. Better still, save such titillating fare for weekends when you can make up for it if you have trouble getting to sleep. During the week, lean toward comedy and music. As for television, the advent of videotape is a great boon to insomniacs. Now you can tape those 10 o'clock dramas and late-night talk shows and watch them at a more appropriate time. Why not try David Letterman in the morning over breakfast after you've had a good night's sleep?

A businessman named Arthur Kaplan always had trouble sleeping on Monday night. For a long time he thought this was because Tuesday was the day of his weekly staff meetings, which he had come to dread. When his meetings were switched to Thursdays, he assumed he'd have trouble sleeping on Wednesdays. Not so. Monday was still the troublesome night. Then he discovered the reason: Monday Night Football. After the games he would toss and turn, replaying all the big plays in his mind's eye. When he decided to limit his football viewing to Sundays, Kaplan slept a whole lot better. (Several insomniac sports fans have admitted to a similar fate with evening spectatorship. They all noticed the same thing: when their team won, they slept well; when their team lost, they lost sleep. We wonder if there are a disproportionate number of insomniacs among Chicago Cub fans.)

Even your conversations can affect your sleep. On week-nights, don't invite guests over with whom you are likely to get into a late-night argument or an especially stimulating discussion that will keep you up thinking after the lights are out. Save those occasions for holidays or weekends. It's also best not to start an argument late at night. If you have a bone to pick with your spouse, pick it early. That will give you time to calm down, and hopefully make up, before going to sleep.

REGULARITY

Almost every authority in the field recommends—and insists on—regular sleeping habits. Experiment and find the most efficient time for you to get to sleep and stick to it. If you find a set of rituals that creates the proper mood and atmosphere for sleep, stick with that too. The repetition will help you gain sleep habits that will eventually become involuntary and effortless.

Once you establish a bedtime, get ready for it well in advance. Joan Black, an insomniac college student who was ordered by her doctor to be in bed by 11, found after two weeks that it had made no difference in the quality of her sleep. It seems she would wait until the last possible moment before dropping her studies or her socializing, then dash into the bathroom, brush her teeth, rush into the bedroom, and quickly undress. She practically dove into bed just under the wire every night, diligently following the letter of the doctor's orders but not really the spirit. It still took her an hour to fall asleep because that's how long she needed to wind down.

It's a good idea to perform your ablutions and rituals early and leisurely. While you are preparing for bed, turn your thoughts to something pleasant. Don't plan the next day's schedule or contemplate its potential problems. Some habitual worriers keep a pad and pencil at their bedsides and write down what's on their minds along with their plans and goals for the next day. They claim that this ritual stops them from ruminating in endless circles. When you write things down, it lends an authority and finality to thoughts that helps stop the worry-go-round.

What time should you go to bed? Obviously, that is an individual matter. If your body does not dictate an unequivocal answer—that is, if you have a choice as to what time to get in bed—it's a good idea to opt for the earlier hour. The old adage about early to bed and early to rise may have more going for it than a catchy rhyme. "One hour's sleep before midnight is worth two after," wrote Henry Fielding, a notion that has been echoed many times. There might be something to it. A study by Australian researchers Johns, Dudley, and Masterson noted that "better academic performance as a medical student has been shown to be related both to early morning awakening and to better mental health."

For a more scientific method of selecting your best sleep time, try going by your temperature. It has been found that a person's body temperature drops at night, and according to one science writer that's a signal to the body that it's time to go to sleep. You might take your temperature a few times during the evening for a few nights to pinpoint the time when it drops.

Probably the best way to determine your maximal opportunity to sleep is simply to listen to the signals from your body. When the yawns come, when the mind starts to wander, when you find yourself reading every paragraph twice or you can't tell the difference between the TV show and the commercials, then it's probably time to shut your eyes for the night. Don't make the mistake—a common one, often a throwback to childhood when we hated to go to bed because we might miss something—of fighting the impulse to sleep. Tape the show, put the book down, postpone the conversation. If you fight to stay awake a little longer you are likely to win—and the effects of that victory will linger.

TIME THERAPY

One of the more promising new treatments developed since the advent of sleep research is *chronotherapy*, or time therapy. Developed by Dr. Elliot Phillips, medical director of the Sleep Disorders Center at Holy Cross Hospital in Mission Hills, California, the treatment involves systematically changing the times you go to bed and awaken until your biological clock is reset and you can sleep when you want to and wake up refreshed when you have to.

Chronotherapy requires strong motivation and dedication to the task, because it involves following strictly what will seem to be a bizarre schedule for about 10 days. Here's how it works: You make a plan calling for you to go to bed two or three hours later every night. Once begun, you set your alarm to wake you up two or three hours later every morning, corresponding to the changes in your sleeptime schedule. You are to follow the schedule no matter how sleepy you are, and no naps are allowed. At first your internal clock will be totally confused, but that is precisely the intention. You have to unset the clock before you can reset it. Eventually, your clock can be shifted to the sleep and wake times you want to keep.

Here is an example of a chronotherapy schedule for an insomniac who was unable to fall asleep until well after midnight and had trouble getting out of bed before noon (the night before beginning the routine she had gone to sleep at 3 A.M. and awakened at 11):

Night 1: Go to bed no earlier than 5 A.M. and get out of bed no later than 1 P.M.

Night 2: Go to bed no earlier than 7 A.M.; get up no later than 3 P.M.

Night 3: Go to bed no earlier than 9 A.M.; get up no later than 5 P.M.

Night 4: Go to bed no earlier than 11 A.M.; get up no later than 7 P.M.

And so forth, until:

Night 9: Go to bed no earlier than 9 P.M.; get up no later than 5 A.M.

Finally, on *Night 10*: Go to bed at the time that is best for you but no earlier than 9 P.M. And no matter what time you go to bed, get up no later than the time you want to get up every morning. The point is to follow the routine diligently until you have rotated around the clock to the schedule you want, or need, to maintain.

Dr. Phillips advises that you schedule your chronotherapy routine around a holiday or sick leave because you will obviously be totally out of sync with your environment during the 10 days. Naturally, you will need the cooperation and support of friends and family or your employer during this experiment. He also cautions that some people have such weak internal rhythms that they need to repeat the chronotherapy before it works.

SNACKS AND NIGHTCAPS

The great actress Marlene Dietrich once said that the only thing that helped her sleep was a sardine-and-onion sandwich on rye. Teddy Roosevelt was lulled to sleep by a shot of cognac in a glass of milk.

We can't say whether or not sardines or cognac will work for you, but we can say that what you eat at night does make a difference. Certain snacks and nightcaps have been said to improve sleep. In the absence of reliable data, we advise you to try those mentioned here—the ones that appeal to your taste buds, of course—and see if any prove soporific.

Earlier, we indicated that sugar, starch, salt, and especially caffeine can adversely affect sleep. If you cannot eliminate those substances entirely, you should at least cut down on them and restrict their intake to the earlier part of the day.

You might also be wary of too much fruit—although terrific for your health, fruit does contain high concentrations of fructose, which is a sugar, and might raise your blood sugar high enough to interfere with sleep.

Nutrition experts who have worked with insomniacs recommend leaning toward protein, calcium, and vitamin B foods at night. Keep your evening meal moderate, because overeating can destroy sleep. At the same time, hunger can keep you up. So find a sensible, happy medium, eat easily digested foods, and aim for getting to bed with a comfortable tummy—neither too full nor too empty.

For your snacks, dairy products such as the standard glass of warm milk might be best. They are rich in both protein and calcium, and often in l-tryptophan as well (low-fat or no-fat dairy products, by the way, sacrifice none of these ingredients and are kinder to your waistline). If you are inclined to crunchier kinds of snacks, try unsalted nuts or sunflower seeds.

Various cultures throughout the world have discovered their own sleep-inducing foods and beverages. Here are some samples:

The Burmese eat pollen cakes at night.

Pueblo Indians eat large amounts of mushrooms (which have lots of B vitamins).

An ancient Chinese prescription for insomnia is to take an extract of chopped ginseng and dried orange peel fortified with honey; it is to be consumed right before going to sleep. (One of the active ingredients in ginseng is saponin, which has been used to treat hypertension.)

An old English favorite is to eat a large apple, chewing it slowly, before going to bed. Also, English farmers shared the following recipe with the Romany Gypsies: Take the outside leaves of a large head of lettuce and put them in a saucepan with half a pint of boiling water. Add salt, simmer for 20 minutes, strain and serve.

Gypsies, whose sleep has to adapt to constantly changing

environments, also make a fruit drink to be taken just before bed. Mix the juice of one lemon and one orange in a glass with two tablespoons of honey. Fill the glass with hot water and drink slowly. Hot grapefruit juice is also used.

From the countryside of Scotland comes this remedy for insomnia: Oatmeal gruel. Fortunately, it is recommended with lots of honey.

The well-rested farmers of Vermont swear by this remedy: Mix three tablespoons of apple cider vinegar with a cupful of honey. At bedtime, swallow two teaspoonfuls. If still awake an hour later, take two more teaspoonfuls and keep doing that until you fall asleep.

Two others that seem unappetizing but are supported by considerable folklore are raw onions and olive oil. No, not together. The raw onions can be eaten on toast at bedtime. The olive oil should be taken after the evening meal and before bed—one teaspoon each time. To better digest this oily remedy, try filling two dessert spoons with malted milk powder and pour them into a mixer with the one teaspoon of olive oil. Add hot water and shake. Drink this no less than an hour before bedtime.

The hardy Balkan mountaineers have an old tradition that might have some basis in scientific fact: Drinking a glass of buttermilk half an hour before bed. Buttermilk is an excellent source of calcium, which is essential for proper sleep.

Then there is the perennial warm milk. The calcium and l-tryptophan make milk attractive, and heating it up may add to its effect because the warmth increases the flow of blood to the abdominal area. This not only aids digestion but also reduces the amount of blood in the head, which is thought to aid sleep. Don't drink the milk too hot. If you like, add a teaspoon of honey or malt powder for taste. Postum or Ovaltine with the warm milk can also work. As a variation on the theme, try Gaylord Hauser's "sleep cocktail": a cup of hot milk with two teaspoons of the darkest molasses you can find. The B vitamins in the molasses add to the sedative effect.

HERBAL REMEDIES

The *Ayurveda,* an Indian encyclopedia on the healing arts, was said to have been composed thousands of years ago when an ancient sage was walking through the forest and the wild herbs sang to him of their curative powers. Around 3000 B.C. in China, the Emperor Shen Ung lauded the glories of several hundred medicinal herbs; these remedies were encoded and are still in use. The clay tablets of ancient Sumerians and Assyrians, 4,500 years old, record the attributes of some 250 herbs. In our own ancient cultural roots, Hippocrates, the father of medicine, extolled the value of herbs and Aristotle classified hundreds of herbs according to their specific effects.

Despite their illustrious past—and despite the fact that many modern pharmaceuticals were derived from plant-based folk remedies—herbs as cures are frowned upon by modern medicine. Many feel that herbal remedies have not been adequately tested and can be harmful. This argument is countered by those who contend that most herbs are safe and have been used for much longer than modern drugs whose safety is dubious at best.

Herbalists, who are not permitted to prescribe remedies because they are not licensed to practice medicine, have nonetheless published the known uses of herbs, many of which are said to have an effective sedative and tranquilizing action with no side effects. Herbs can be obtained in many health-food stores or in herbalist shops, and of course many can be grown in your own garden.

In addition to the Chinese herbs mentioned in chapter 4, here are some herbal teas that are said to be effective for sleep:

The natives of the West Indies drink *passion flower* tea before retiring.

The Hopi Indians use several herbs to bring on sleep, the most effective being *sand verbena,* a tall, straggling herb with papery fruits that grows in abundance in the mesas of the

Southwest. The Hopi use it especially for helping their children sleep.

Catnip is said to be an effective sedative that quickly brings on drowsiness and a deep, natural sleep. We had a first-hand verification of this when a friend was shaken up in a minor automobile accident. She was unable to settle down, so we served her a cup of catnip tea. Half an hour later she felt too sleepy to drive home.

Lime blossom tea is recommended as a harmless, pleasant bedtime drink because the mineral traces it contains are said to be soothing to the nervous system. To add to its effectiveness, mix in a pinch of *skullcap*.

A nice combination drink that many have found helpful consists of a spoonful each of *valerian*, catnip, skullcap, and hops in a pint of boiling water. Let it steep for 15 minutes and drink shortly before bedtime. (Valerian by itself is commonly recommended for insomnia; its sedative effects have been time-tested.)

Primrose tea is recommended for hypersensitive people and for those who are high-strung and restless in bed.

For general nervousness, *rhododendron*, or "snowrose," is suggested.

Those who have nightmares have been encouraged to drink a combination of *peony* and *spurge laurel*.

For twitching muscles as well as dizziness and headaches that interfere with sleep, the choice seems to be *hops*. Hops is said to be rich in B vitamins, which has long been an excuse for ale drinking in England.

The granddaddy of all sleep-inducing herbs is *chamomile*. This sweet, fragrant flower has been used for centuries as a safe, strong sedative. It is easy to obtain in tea-bag form at any health-food store and at many supermarkets now that large companies such as Lipton and Bigelow are marketing herbal teas.

Chamomile's sedative effects had unexpected verification from science in the 1970s. A team led by Dr. Lawrence Gould was running a series of tests to see if chamomile had any

effect on the cardiac conditions of patients who had under-
gone ventricular catheterizations. It had none. But the scientists were astonished to find a different reaction. In the
Journal of Clinical Pharmacology, Gould wrote: "A striking
hypnotic action of the tea was noted in ten of the twelve patients. It is most unusual for patients undergoing cardiac
catheterizations to fall asleep. The anxiety produced by this
procedure as well as the pain associated with cardiac catheterizations all but preclude sleep. Thus, the fact that ten out of
twelve patients fell into a deep slumber shortly after drinking
chamomile tea is all the more striking."

If that isn't enough of an endorsement, consider that Elizabeth Taylor—who usually sleeps only four or five hours a
night—drinks a blend of chamomile and mint teas so she can
get the eight hours she'd prefer.

Finally, some of the leading tea companies produce
brands with the stated purpose of aiding sleep. The original,
Celestial Seasonings' "Sleepytime" tea, has been followed by
similar recipes by other companies with names such as "Sandman" and "Dream Time." Each of these contains chamomile
as the principal ingredient, and adds spearmint, lemongrass,
blackberry, rosebuds, and other herbs to create a soothing,
tasteful mix.

For more information on herbs, consult one of the follow-
ing books: *The Herb Book,* by John Lust; *Medical Botany,* by
Walter Lewis and Memory Elvin-Lewis; *Mastering Herbalism,*
by Paul Huson; *Herbs and Things,* by Jeanne Rose; *Herbs to
Put You to Sleep,* by Ceres; and the classic *Back to Eden,* by
Jethro Kloss.

YOUR BEDROOM ENVIRONMENT

On seeing a newspaper ad for 600 sleep-aid products, the irrepressible Ogden Nash wrote a poem cataloging the slumber
buzzer, the eyeshade, the snore ball, and the electric slippers,
and asked how our ancestors were able to sleep so well with-

out such gizmos. His point is well-taken—there should be no need for all the various gadgets that have been invented for insomniacs.

Everyone likes a new toy, but sometimes we moderns rely on gadgets so much that we forget how to rely on ourselves. Remember, therefore, as we discuss the accoutrements of the optimal environment for sleep, that *you* are your own best ally in the fight against sleeplessness. Your goal should be self-sufficiency. That is, your mind and body should be so well tuned that you are able to fall asleep when you are tired. Nonetheless, the environment does make a difference and ought to be considered an integral part of a holistic approach to sleep.

For much of our information on the sleeper's environment, we called on the man who has been called America's Public Sandman, Norman Dine. An insomniac, he sold his furniture business in the 1930s and set out to learn all he could about sleep. When, eventually, he conquered his own insomnia, Dine combined his new expertise with his knowledge of the furniture business and became America's first bona fide sleep merchant. His shop in New York, and later in New Jersey, became a haven for insomniacs and the prototype for many imitations around the country.

Dine used to divide human beings into two categories: the "constitutionally fortunate" and "light sleepers." The former have no need for sleep aids; the latter need all the help they can get in warding off irritants such as noise, light, pressure, heat, cold, drafts, stuffiness, humidity, a restless spouse, and other sleep-robbers. Drawing on Dine and other experts, the following pages discuss various aspects of the bedroom environment and various accessories that you might look into.

The Sounds of Slumber

When poet Amy Lowell stayed in a hotel, she would rent five rooms—one to sleep in, one empty room on each side, and one above and below. She simply could not tolerate noise.

Sleep specialists would probably say that Lowell was so sensitive to noise because she was a poor sleeper, not vice versa. Nonetheless, noise can be a sleep-stealing nuisance.

We know that some sounds have a soothing, lulling, restful effect. When we need repose, we seek the quiet sounds of the woods, the rain, gentle music, or the somnolent melody of waves lapping a shore. When we want to guide our babies gently into sleep, we hum lullabies. Yet we also know the effects of other sounds, such as Sousa marches. Sousa we use when we want to stir the mind and soul to action with rousing drumbeats and trumpets. And if we ever get the urge to drive our fellow creatures out of their minds, we use harsh, jarring, dissonant sounds such as heavy-metal music. Sometimes we literally drive ourselves crazy, as in the case of the French factory workers who suddenly began complaining of nausea, fatigue, and irritability for no apparent reason. It was later discovered that recently installed machinery produced sounds that were, although beyond the range of human hearing, upsetting the workers' nervous systems.

The autonomic nervous system, which controls involuntary activities such as the heartbeat, begins to react to sounds at 70 decibels. Sounds above that threshold, especially those that are irregular, unpredictable, and meaningless, raise the blood pressure and cut down the supply of blood to the heart. As the intensity of the noise increases, the emergencylike response gets more severe: pupils dilate, mouth and tongue get dry, muscles contract, heartbeat quickens, adrenaline pours forth. There is some indication that exposure to high-volume noise raises the likelihood of heart attacks.

Unfortunately, the sounds in the air when we try to go to sleep are often in the high-decibel range. The traffic on a relatively quiet city street is approximately 70 decibels, just about the level at which the autonomic nervous system begins to respond. And it responds when we are asleep as well. Even if the sounds do not wake you up or prevent you from falling asleep, the slight arousal they elicit can prevent you from getting the most beneficial sleep.

What to do? You can move to the countryside for one thing, but that is not always convenient. Nor is it always quiet. Superhighways, televisions, stereos, trucks, motorcycles, and teenagers are everywhere.

One solution is to use earplugs. There are several good brands on the market. The type designed to keep water out of the ears of swimmers is not recommended for noise. Plugs made of soft, malleable wax that can be molded to cover the outer part of the ear without having to be pressed too deeply into the opening are effective, except the wax tends to rub off. This means you have to replace them fairly often (we know someone in New York City who wears them every night; he goes through a box every two months). It also means that some of the wax might rub off in your ear. Although that seems to be easily remedied by soap and water, we do not know what effects there might be if the wax oozes down the ear canal.

Our personal favorite is the Noise Filter, manufactured by the E-A-R Group, a division of the Cabot Corporation in Indianapolis. Made of soft foam, the plugs feature a time-delayed expansion. You compress one, roll it into a narrow cylinder, and insert it into the ear opening. The plug then expands to a snug fit that conforms to the shape of your ear canal. Reusable and safe, the filters are effective enough to be widely used by workers in noisy factories and by regular subway riders in New York. They are very inexpensive and are available in most large drugstores.

Earplugs will muffle any sound that comes along, but they can't eliminate all noise entirely. Moreover, some people do not like total silence, preferring sleep-encouraging sounds instead. What do you do if gentle raindrops, soothing wind, or rolling surf is unavailable when you want to sleep? You can buy an electronic *sound conditioner*, such as the Sleep Coaxer, for one thing. This handy little device (it weighs only two pounds) masks out disturbing noises with the drowsing sounds of surf, rain, or wind.

Also available is Marpac Company's Sleep-Mate, which

creates an adjustable, windlike sound. Compact and portable, the device has been tested at a major sleep laboratory and found to be harmless. It does not interfere with normal sleep cycles. Like the Sleep Coaxer, it is designed for continuous operation and consumes no more electricity than a small night-light.

That certain sounds can foster slumber has been verified by hundreds of stories of people who can't get to sleep without their favorites, whether a roaring river (which might keep cityfolk awake) or the ticking of a grandfather clock. Most of us know someone who falls asleep with the TV or radio on only to wake with a start when someone shuts it off. Scientists have found that newborn infants can be lulled to sleep with recordings that simulate their mothers' heartbeats.

The advantage of sound conditioners is that, in most cases, they have been constructed to provide a bland, low-frequency sound that blends with others and can modify even sharp and unexpected noises, thus reducing the severity of their impact. The extremes are less extreme and therefore less annoying.

A breaking-in period may be needed with these devices. Some insomniacs report having stopped using theirs because they irritated them. Those who stuck it out soon became used to the new sound and in most cases found their sleep improved. If you have trouble breaking in your sound machine, start by using it for a short period of time before going to bed. Gradually increase the amount of time you use it and the volume setting. Soon the sound will become part of the background and you will forget it is present.

Many people think that friendly sounds are useless unless they completely block out other noise. This is not so. To do that the sound would have to be louder than the loudest harmful sound, and that, in itself, would be harmful. The intention is simply to mask or nullify existing sounds.

Specialty shops or mail-order catalogs such as Sharper Image offer sound-producing devices of varying sophistication and cost. An alternative, of course, is to purchase tapes or

compact discs of nature sounds; these come in several varieties, from rain forests to deserts. You could even make a tape
of the sounds that you find most sleep-conducive. Then again,
if your needs are best served by a constant, neutral sound, you
may need to do nothing more than run your fan or air-
conditioner and let the hum lull you to sleep.

Of all the available sound sources for insomniacs, perhaps
the most time-tested is music. In the eighteenth century a
young prince suffering from severe sleeplessness asked his
protégé, a young musician named Goldberg, to help him overcome his problem. Goldberg took the request to his music
teacher, who composed a slow, enchanting piece of piano music for the prince. The composer was Johann Sebastian Bach,
and the composition became known as *The Goldberg Variations*. It worked for the prince, and you might find it soothing
too, particularly in recordings of solo piano.

We asked several musicians and music experts to recommend "music to fall asleep by." The variety of responses was
astonishing; one person's noise was another's lullaby. Most
leaned toward nonsymphonic classical music, principally by
soloists and small chamber groups. Music with lyrics or pronounced rhythmic accents were felt to be arousing or likely to
draw too much attention to itself.

The pieces most frequently mentioned: Brahms' "Lullaby,"
Schubert's "Serenade," Debussy's "Afternoon of a Faun" and
"Girl with Flaxen Hair," Mozart quartets, Chopin nocturnes,
and guitar and harp solos. You could also try the Wyndham
Hill recordings of pianist George Winston. In addition, there
are now dozens of New Age recordings written and arranged
expressly to relax and soothe. The range of choice in this
category is enormous, but one album worth a listen is *Lullabies and Sweet Dreams*, serene improvisations on familiar
themes such as "Twinkle, Twinkle, Little Star" and Brahms'
"Lullaby." This is part of the Anti-Frantic Alternative series
from the catalog of Sound Rx, P.O. Box 1439, San Rafael, CA
94915.

With a little trial and error, you should be able to put together a personal sleep-enhancing music library.

In the Dark

Most of us have experienced trying to fall asleep in a room with too much light. Like noise, light is stimulating, and closing your eyes is not enough; some light finds its way through. Studies have shown that even the activity level of the kidneys increases and decreases according to the amount of light in a room, so it is no wonder that the sleep mechanism is likewise affected.

The solution: good window shades and thick drapes, and if that's not enough, eyeshades. We have found that a good eyeshade can effectively keep out virtually all light rays. It may take a night or two to get used to having a shade against your face, but soon enough it will become part of your bedroom milieu. A well-designed shade can be worn fairly loose without reducing its effectiveness. The better brands are black (at least on the side facing your eyes), have a soft, satiny texture, and contain light padding for the bridge of the nose.

What if you don't like total darkness or can't sleep in a completely dark room? If you require *some* light, make sure it's soft and indirect. Or, purchase what's been called the "claustrophobic's eyeshade." It has tiny pinholes that admit a small amount of subdued light.

Finally, if you like a dark room but sleep with a spouse who stays up to read, consult catalogs and specialty shops for a reading lamp that projects a clear, nonglaring beam. According to a brochure for one such product, "It leaves you in soothing darkness and lets him finish the chapter."

Bedding Down

O bed! O bed! Delicious bed!
That heaven on earth to the weary head!
THOMAS HOOD

We spend over one third of our lives in our beds, so we owe it to ourselves to have the right kind of habitat. Just what "right" is varies with each individual, however. Queen Esther, the first person in the Bible whose bed is mentioned, slept on a bunch of cushions flung into a corner. Emperor Nero's bed was a little more ornate; it was encrusted with precious stones alleged to have beneficial powers—rubies, amethysts, garnets, and diamonds. Finicky Louis XIV of France owned 413 beds, enough to sleep in a different one every night of the year with an extra one for every weekend. And Benjamin Franklin, a fanatic for cool-air slumber, reportedly kept four beds in his room so that he could rotate as each one became warm.

Perhaps the first bed question we should address is the delicate one of single versus double beds. Among married insomniacs the issue frequently comes up in the offices of marriage counselors. Dr. P. J. Steincrohn recommends twin beds for restless-sleeping couples: "There is more likelihood of loss of sleep and consequent irritability and argument in double beds than in twin beds (no elbows in the ribs, no twisting and turning)."

If, as a couple, your preferences for bedroom conditions are irreconcilable, you might consider the seemingly drastic step of sleeping in separate rooms—or at least be prepared for that contingency at certain times, such as when one person is exceptionally restless or in the case of severe snoring (about which more later on). It might seem unromantic to split up the marriage bed that way, but better the bed than the marriage. We are never more irrational or pugnacious than when we are tired and someone else—no matter how beloved—disturbs our sleep.

If you do choose mutual exile, don't fret. Think of how romantic a surprise visit can be. "My bed or yours?"

Your mattress.   Most back specialists advocate the use of a firm mattress. Orthopedist Leon Root, coauthor of *Oh, My Aching Back*, says that a hard foam mattress, 4 to 6 inches thick on a platform foundation or a 1-inch thick plywood board, is the best thing for an aching back. Firm mattresses, he says, "tend to keep the lower back from sagging."

However, many people are sleeping on mattresses that are actually *too* firm for their own good. A mattress should fit your individual needs—your height, weight, shape, posture, sleep pattern, sensitivity to pressure, the length and curvature of your back, and other factors should all be considered.

As a rule, a light sleeper should avoid as many irritants as possible. For example, your mattress should be 8 to 10 inches longer than your height and 7 to 10 inches wider than you are. If you *literally* slept like a log—that is, if you didn't move—that extra room would not be necessary. But even the most loglike sleepers change position about 20 times a night, and some of us change 50 times or more. We need space to maneuver comfortably.

All that movement makes the quality of your mattress that much more important. Moving around changes the parts of the body that are subject to pressure and redistributes the flow of circulation. If your bed is too soft or too hard your *motility* (spontaneous movements) will be restricted.

Here are some guidelines with which to evaluate your mattress:

If there is painful pressure at the heavier parts of your body such as the hips, if your sleeping positions seem insecure and the number of positions you can assume are limited, if there is coolness under your body, then your mattress is probably *too firm*.

Thin people, whose bones are not well-cushioned, and people with curvatures of the spine usually need more resiliency and less firmness; a hard mattress will press excessively against parts of your body.

If you have back fatigue or a sagging spine, if you feel undue body warmth or a swaying sensation and restricted movement, chances are your mattress is *too soft*.

Look for effortless buoyancy, a cradling sensation, even

support, complete freedom of movement, and gentle pressure evenly distributed throughout your whole body. Says Dr. W. W. Bauer, "The best condition for good sleep is gentle support of the body at all points, and without permitting too much lateral bending of the spine."

When mattress shopping, always lie down on the mattress. Don't just push and prod; stretch out and relax on it. Hunt around. Find one that feels just right, keeping in mind such factors as buoyancy, resilience, and silence (no squeaking springs). Look for lots of quilting, and an inner spring unit with a coil count of at least 300 for every 54 inches of mattress. Don't be carried away by pretty designs. Also, look for a long warranty. Remember that although a smooth surface may look more attractive, the tufted mattress is better and will retain its shape longer without sagging. Check beyond the name of the model; some manufacturers call identical mattresses by different names so they can be sold at different prices. Bear in mind also that many people prefer the firmness, convenience, and moderate pricing of futons.

Once you purchase a mattress, treat it well so it will give you maximum service over time. Break it in correctly. During the first six months of use, turn it over and end to end once a month. After that do it twice a year. Once a month air out the mattress with the windows open and vacuum it thoroughly— even the box spring. Always use a mattress pad.

Another factor to keep in mind is allergies. Many people are allergic to the kapok used to stuff some mattresses. Others are allergic to foam, horsehair, or feathers. Such allergies, says Dr. Claude A. Frazier, afflict 15 to 20 percent of the population. If you find yourself coughing or wheezing at night, if you have headaches or snore excessively, and if you have dark circles under your eyes even when rested, you might be allergic to your mattress. Dr. Frazier recommends rigorous vacuuming of mattresses to keep out the dust, which is a common irritant. And wrap everything in allergen-proof protective covers and tape up the zippers.

If you are interested in the luxury of a bed that adjusts to a variety of head, back, and leg angles and also provides electric massage at the touch of a button, contact Ultra-Bed, 39337 Ide Court, Fremont, CA 94538.

Your pillow.   Traditional Japanese rest their heads on blocks of wood. Zulus also sleep on wood, delicately carved. In czarist Russia children were given elegant little pillows trimmed with lace, called *doumkas*—literally, "the one you tell your thoughts to."

We have no such quaint customs, but what we rest our heads on influences our sleep nonetheless. Pillows should be just thick enough to hold the head in the same relation to the shoulders and spine that it has when we stand up. One way to test this is to stand sideways with your shoulder touching a wall. Place the pillow on your shoulder. It should fit perfectly between the head and the wall without your bending your neck.

If your pillow is too thick it can strain the neck muscles. If your head sinks too deeply into the pillow it can cause overheating and make changing positions more difficult. In addition, the strain on the shoulder and neck muscles can cut off circulation, causing "pins and needles" in the arms and hands, or other discomforts that can keep you awake. There is no scientific evidence to support the theory that raising the head to drain blood from it, or lowering the head to increase blood flow to it—each of which has been lauded as beneficial to sleep—has any validity.

Experts say that sleeping on your side in the manner described in chapter 9 is ideal. However, it takes a long time for anyone to learn new sleep positions, and we tend to shift back into habitual positions in our sleep. If you find yourself sleeping on your back, a position that is not recommended, you might want to try a cigar-shaped pillow filled with a soft, malleable filling. A good one will adjust to the contours of your neck, cradling it and protecting the neck muscles, which can get seriously damaged from sleeping on your back on the wrong pillow—try Dr. Jackson's Neck Pillow.

The trouble with most pillows is that they do not respect the contours of the body. Someone once made them box-shaped and box-shaped they remained. Several manufacturers have designed contour pillows that elevate the head without irritating the shoulders or neck. Check out the products of the following companies: Jantz Design and Manufacturing, P.O. Box 3071, Santa Rosa, CA 95402; and Sobagara Enterprises, Inc., 1630 Liholiho St., Honolulu, HI 96822.

Well-stocked shops carry a variety of pillows for special purposes—everything from pillows that raise the head or feet for those with particular breathing or circulation problems, to foam bolster pillows in wedgelike shapes for sitting up and reading or placing under your knees (many people find their circulation greatly aided by having their knees elevated).

Most pillows nowadays are made of synthetic materials, which are better for allergy sufferers. The best is said to be "continuous multifilament fiber." It is spun into the casing, comes in a wide range of different degrees of firmness, and does not shift, settle, or wad up. Synthetics last for about 5 to 7 years. Goose-down pillows are lusciously comfortable, and with proper care can last 25 years or more. Since down is very expensive, most feather pillows also include duck, chicken, or turkey feathers, which also provide extra body.

Sheets and blankets.   There is no end to the variety of sheets and blankets now available; they come in all conceivable materials and colors. If you can afford it, silk is still the preferred choice, probably because of its softness. Cotton (100 percent) is next best, because its natural texture has none of the discomfort and creates less of the static electricity that comes from rubbing against synthetics. Generally speaking, you should select a material that feels pleasant to the touch and does not offend any allergies you may have.

As for color, the choice may be more than aesthetic. There is some evidence that the effects of color, though largely unconscious, can be profound. One manufacturer suggests pastels or neutral colors, such as beige, for those whose days are hectic, and deep, bold colors for those whose days are dull. Louis Cheskin of the Color Research Institute of America says that red has a violently stimulating effect, whereas blue, the coolest of all colors, is said to be a sedative with the capacity to soothe mental agitation. Scandinavian physicist Oscar Brunler once suggested that all poor sleepers should use pale blue sheets and sleep in blue pajamas. "If you are a poor sleeper," he wrote, "visualize blue all around you."

Greens also are said to be calming. It is well-known that green is the most soothing light vibration—one reason, perhaps, why the lush green of the countryside makes us feel so good.

These factors may seem trivial, and relatively speaking they probably are, but if you are not sleeping well you can use all the help you can get. So why not consider a color change for sheets, and maybe even for wallpaper, paint, and pajamas as well?

The important thing about sheets is that they be clean, smooth, and cool. The top sheet should fit rather loosely at the foot (for some reason, we tend to make our beds in such a way that our feet are inhibited). Your feet should have room to maneuver, so they will not get cramped and wake you up.

Blankets are a less trivial concern. A study by General Electric revealed that differences as small as 1 degree higher or lower in bed temperature made a noticeable difference in the quality of sleep. How heavily a sleeper should be blanketed is an individual matter, having to do largely with the discharge of body heat. Those who lose a great deal of heat need heavier covering than those who hold sufficient heat on their own.

Electric blankets ideally should be thermostatically controlled to respond to the temperature of the body as it changes. Such a blanket was actually produced and worked perfectly—in the laboratory; for some reason, it never worked in the hands of consumers. So thermostats in commercial electric blankets respond to the temperature of the room, not the body. This is satisfactory but not ideal, and many health experts question whether encasing yourself in an electric current for eight hours is a smart idea.

Whatever they are made of, your blankets should not be too heavy. Consider that in eight hours of sleep you lift your bedclothes at least 7,000 times by breathing. In addition to electric blankets, eiderdown comforters and various kinds of quilts can provide excellent insulation without weighing you down. Experiment to find the best cover for you. You can even buy an automatic bed warmer that fits between the mattress and the sheets to provide warmth from beneath you in winter. You might also check out the Jantz Company's lambswool mattress pad, which they say keeps you cooler when you are hot and warms you up quickly when you are cold.

The Temperature and the Air You Breathe

Benjamin Franklin (who had four beds in his room) lived to be 84 years old at a time when the life expectancy was only 35. Perhaps one reason was his ability to sleep soundly. Here is his prescription:

> When you are waked up by uneasiness, and find you cannot sleep easily again, get out of bed, beat up and turn up your pillow, shake the bed clothes well with at least twenty shakes, then throw the bed open and leave it to cool; in the meanwhile, continuing undressed, walk about your chamber, till your skin has had time to discharge its load, which it will do sooner, as the air may be drier and colder.
>
> When you begin to feel the cold air unpleasant, then return to your bed; you will soon fall asleep, and your sleep will be sweet and pleasant.

It is hard to say whether it was the freshness of the air or its coolness that helped Mr. Franklin sleep. Both, however, are said to be important.

The ideal temperature for sound sleep is between 64° and 66° Fahrenheit. Sleep researchers have found that people tend to need more sleep when the bedroom temperature is lower than 60° and are less likely to sleep long enough to feel rested if the bedroom temperature is above 70°. Although the main concern is your individual comfort (which just might require a temperature outside the range mentioned above), most experts seem to lean toward cooler temperatures.

If your blanket warms all of your body except your feet, try wearing heavy socks. Charles Darwin rarely slept without them. If you need something more, sporting goods stores and camping supply houses sell a wide variety of light, unobtrusive feet warmers, made of goose down and other material. Or you can purchase an electric warming pad that goes under your sheet to keep your feet warm by thermostatic control.

In hot weather, air conditioning is useful, of course, although many people complain about the artificiality of the air and prefer to use a fan. Sometimes a cool top sheet is more comfortable, even on the hottest nights, than no top sheet at all. Avoid the temptation of cooling off with a cold shower before bed. It will stimulate your body to produce more heat.

Hot, congested head and eyes can cause sleeplessness. Bathe the eyes with cold water and use a cold-water compress on the eyelids and forehead before going to bed. The compress is a traditional balm used in the Middle East, where they know how to deal with hot, dry air.

As for ventilation, there is some debate about the ideal conditions. Common sense and most experts argue against stuffy rooms, but others point out that it is in those very stuffy rooms that we tend to get drowsy. Watch what happens in a conference room in the winter when the windows are closed. The advocates of stuffy bedrooms say that if you air out the room before bed, take in a few deep breaths of air, and have reasonably healthy lungs, you will have all the air you need with plenty to spare. Dr. Charles Kelly, whose breathing method we describe in chapter 9, demonstrated that two sleeping people cannot use up enough air in an ordinary-sized bedroom for either to notice the difference.

Then there is the story of that classic fresh-air fiend, Ben Franklin. Once he had to share a room with a man who could not sleep with the window open. As might be expected, Franklin won the ensuing debate and the shutters were opened wide. Franklin slept perfectly and his poor roommate did not sleep a wink. But in the morning, they discovered that the shutters they had opened onto the fresh night air had actually opened onto a small closet.

Is the answer to the ventilation debate, "It's all in the mind"?

YOGA: STRETCHING INTO THE NIGHT

Vigorous exercise right before bed may be overstimulating, but the more gentle variety that emphasizes stretching has a lot to offer. The authors and many other insomniacs have found Yoga to be exceptionally calming.

The science of Yoga dates back thousands of years to its roots in ancient India. In the West, it was regarded as the province of eccentrics and mystics until recent years when many Americans discovered its value and medical science recognized its health-promoting qualities. Yoga can have an overall normalizing effect on the nervous system and on key organs and glands.

One entire branch of Yoga—the one most familiar to us—specializes in physical exercises. Done correctly, these are more like postures and movements than exercises; they are simple and nonstrenuous. Typically done in the morning to prepare the body and mind for a day of energetic activity, they can also be done at night if you choose the appropriate exercises and perform them correctly.

Ideally, you should learn Yoga from a qualified teacher, either privately or in a class. In lieu of that, there are a number of excellent books and tapes from which you can learn effectively and safely. For our purposes, we will discuss a few exercises that are recommended for insomnia.

Ordinarily, a full set of exercises is not advised for use at night—they would be too energizing. Done correctly, however, certain postures will help you get rid of the stress and tension that keep you awake. Some of these bend and twist the spine, thus freeing the flow of energy. Others loosen and relax various muscles and joints where tension is stored. They also give a valuable inner massage to vital organs such as the liver, kidneys, and stomach, and their soothing influence on the nervous system can help restore the body's natural biorhythms.

Yoga is especially good for people with sedentary jobs. Inactivity can devitalize the body and render it sluggish. These exercises will stimulate proper circulation and help eliminate the free-floating anxiety that can keep you awake when you want to be asleep.

First, some general points to keep in mind when doing Yoga. These are not the kind of exercises we are used to in the West; they should not raise the metabolism or cause exertion. They are meant to conserve, not use, energy. It is very important to perform the movements slowly, gently, and comfortably. Never strain and never force your body into any position that is painful.

The postures as illustrated might look impossible—and for most beginners they are. Few of us have bent, twisted, and stretched in the manner called for. However, it does not matter whether you achieve the position illustrated. What matters is that you move slowly and easily in the direction of the final posture and stop when you begin to feel the strain. Hold the position at that point and consider it done. Gradually, the body will become more flexible. The important thing is the movement itself, not achieving any goal. Straining to bend an extra inch will get you nothing but a pulled muscle, and that is sure to keep you awake.

Wear loose-fitting clothing and practice in a quiet, dimly lit room on a thick carpet or blanket.

The Cobra. This posture promotes relaxation, particularly in the upper back and neck. It stretches and firms the muscles supporting the spine, and stimulates several important organs. It is especially popular among people who bend over a desk all day.

Lie with your arms at your sides with your forehead touching the floor. Slowly, tilt your head back. Using your back muscles, raise your trunk as far off the floor as possible without using your hands. Pretending to try to see as far behind your head as you can, lift first your head, then your neck, shoulders, and back. Now place your hands beneath the shoulders and push up gently and slowly. (See Figure 8-1.) You should feel your back stretch one vertebra at a time.

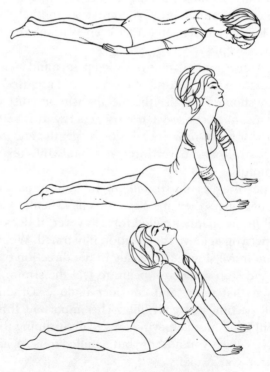

Figure 8-1. The Cobra.

Remember, this is not a push-up. Your arms should not be doing much work; they are used primarily for support while your back muscles do the lifting.

Raise yourself up as far as you can without straining. In the extreme position the arms are straight and the head is tilted far back. The legs should be relaxed throughout, not tensed up. Hold the position that you have comfortably attained for about 10 seconds.

Keeping your spine arched, begin to lower yourself by reversing the procedure. The neck and head should straighten out last, with the forehead returning to touch the floor. Then bring your arms back to your sides and turn your head so that your cheek rests comfortably on the floor. Let your body go limp.

You can repeat this movement two or three times, always doing it slowly and easily, stopping each lift when you begin to feel a strain. Breathe normally throughout.

Neck Twist. The neck area is very vulnerable to tension, especially for those who are sedentary. Look around you at your office and see all the people contorting their necks to relieve the stiffness. Those spontaneous twists are imprecise and haphazard. The following exercise should help you safely relieve tension.

Do this in a relaxed manner with your eyes closed. Make no attempt to crack your neck with sudden or forceful movements. Simply turn as far as possible, stopping when you feel a strain, and hold for about 10 seconds.

Begin by placing your elbows on a level surface—the floor, a table, or a desk. Your arms should be parallel and your elbows fairly close together as you place your head between your hands.

Clasp your hands on the lower part of the back of your head. Don't clasp your neck. Now gently push down until your chin touches your chest. Make sure your elbows are close together so you have enough height to move your head downward. Hold for about 10 seconds.

Turn your head slowly and rest your chin in your left hand so that the fingers rest on your left cheek. Grip the back of your head firmly with your right hand. Now turn your head slowly to the left as far as possible. (See Figure 8-2.) Hold for 10 seconds.

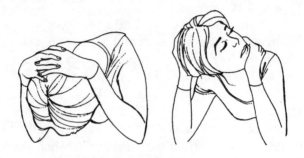

Figure 8-2. Neck Twist.

Now, turn your head slowly to the right and rest your chin in your right palm. This time the fingers should rest along the right cheek. Grip the back of your head firmly with your left hand. Again, turn the head as far as possible, this time to the right, slowly. Hold the position for about 10 seconds.

Remember in doing these neck twists that you want to turn your head as far as it will go without strain. For this you should use your hands to get that extra twist—without yanking or pulling your neck.

Alternate Leg Pulls. Sit with your legs stretched out before you. Place the right heel firmly against the inside of your left thigh. Reach up, lean backward slightly, and then bend forward, taking a firm hold on your left leg or ankle—or, if you are flexible enough, your foot. Now, keeping your back straight, gently pull your trunk downward without straining. You should bend from the hip, not the middle of the back.

With your head limp, move in the direction of touching your forehead to your knee. (See Figure 8-3.) More likely than not, long before your head touches your knee, you will feel a strain in the back of your outstretched leg, in the hamstring muscle, and perhaps also in your back. Hold it right there. Don't attempt to stretch beyond the point of strain.

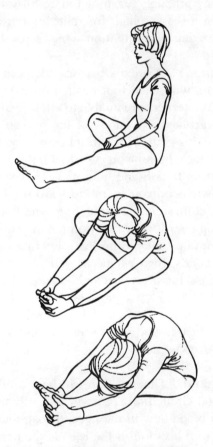

Figure 8-3. Alternate Leg Pulls.

Hold at your point of maximum stretch for about 30 seconds, or less if it becomes uncomfortable. Then repeat the movement with your right leg outstretched. Repeat the series two or three times.

Remember when doing the leg pull that you should grasp your outstretched leg as far forward as is comfortable. For some, that means the toes or the middle of the foot; for others it might mean the shin or even the knee. If your leg tends to lift up, you are probably reaching too far forward.

This posture is excellent for relieving tension in the legs and for improving leg circulation, a big factor in insomnia.

Yoga Mudra.   Yoga adepts perform this one seated in the lotus position, with each foot nestled on the opposite thigh. Since most Westerners are unable to attain that position without tearing cartilage or tendons, ordinary cross-legged seating will do. Sit with your back straight and your arms relaxed behind your back, holding one wrist with the other hand.

Take a deep breath and hold it. Then, keeping your back straight, slowly bend your trunk forward until your forehead touches—or comes close to touching—the floor. As in other postures, stop your forward motion the instant you feel strain or pain. Maintain that posture, still holding your breath, for about 10 seconds, then exhale as you return to the upright position. Pause for a few seconds, take a deep breath, and repeat.

Doing this a few times can be remarkably relaxing. For many people, cares and woes seem to disappear in the few seconds the exercise takes.

Shoulder Stand.   This position will have a noticeable effect on your blood circulation. You will instantly feel a sensation of increased blood flow in the neck, throat, and head, as well as a feeling of relaxation in the legs as the pressure of blood being held down by the force of gravity is relieved. Reversing your body in this way allows a rich supply of blood to enter the regions above the heart, especially the brain. The posture offers a variety of benefits *if you do it correctly*.

Lie on your back with your arms at your sides. Brace the

palms against the floor, stiffen your abdomen and leg muscles, and slowly raise your legs. When your legs are upright, perpendicular to your body, swing them toward your head so your hips leave the floor and prop your hands beneath your hips. Bend your knees if it helps, and then straighten up slowly. You might find it easiest to remain in a position with your hips up and legs bent over your head. (See Figure 8-4.) If you can, straighten up further than this, but please do not be in a hurry to do so. You will get the most out of this exercise by being conservative.

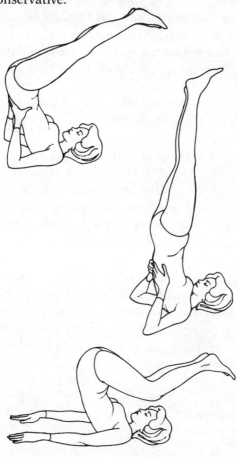

Figure 8-4. Shoulder Stand.

In the completed shoulder stand the legs are absolutely straight and the chin presses against the chest. The body should not be rigid, it should be relaxed, and *the weight should not be on your head or neck* or you risk damaging the upper neck vertebrae. Your shoulders, upper back, and supporting hands should bear the weight. Hold the position for a maximum of 30 seconds.

Coming out of the shoulder stand is as important as going in. Be careful not to collapse out of it; don't crash to the floor. *Bend your knees* and lower your legs slowly. Place your hands at your side for support. Then roll forward slowly and carefully, lowering your hips. When your buttocks touch the floor, hold there, then straighten out your legs and slowly lower them to the floor. Allow your body to go limp and rest for a while.

Once again, do this exercise very carefully. If you are too eager to achieve a perfect shoulder stand you can easily strain your neck.

If you find it too difficult to do the shoulder stand, a good alternative is the use of a slant board. Many sporting and fitness shops sell these. They come with straps or bars to hook your feet under, and they fold up for storage. In addition, you might look into gravity boots and orthopedic swings—in both devices you can easily relax upside down.

Corpse Pose.   Despite its rather morbid name, this pose is everyone's favorite. You simply lie face up, hands at your sides, and relax completely. (See Figure 8-5.) It is a perfect way to end your Yoga routine after coming down from the Shoulder Stand. Keep your palms up and your heels together. Relax.

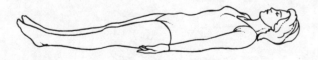

Figure 8-5. Corpse Pose.

Without straining your mind or forcing your body, direct your attention successively to each muscle group in your body. First, feel the tips of your toes, then slowly move your attention up your legs to the feet, ankles, calves, knees, and thighs. Just let your mind fall easily where you direct it without attempting to concentrate or to drive away other thoughts. As you draw the attention to each area, simply let the muscles relax. You might feel them twitch or tense up or even quiver. Just let them find their repose naturally.

From your thighs, continue up your torso to the pelvic area, the stomach, the waist, the chest, the shoulders, then down to your fingers, your hands, your forearms, your biceps, your shoulders. Now, up to the throat and neck, and finally to the face and head. At each stop, linger until that area feels relaxed. When you reach the top of your head, gently shift your attention to the whole body.

By now you might be so relaxed you fall asleep on the floor. For that reason, it might not be a bad idea to do your Yoga in the bedroom.

Long Swing. An astounding amount of tension gets deposited in the muscles around the eyes. Much of the day we strain and overstimulate our eyes; 86 percent of our sensory input is said to be visual. Although not Yoga, the following exercise, developed by ophthalmologist W. H. Bates and lauded by Aldous Huxley in *The Art of Seeing*, will relax your eye muscles and prevent you from "staring" in your dreams, a phenomenon that is said to cause headaches and eyestrain at night.

Stand with your feet comfortably apart and sway slowly from one foot to the other, lifting the heel of one foot when your weight is on the other. Let your arms hang loosely and keep your head straight with your nose pointed straight ahead. Then begin to turn your body in an arc, swinging a full 180 degrees from right to left and back again, allowing hips, shoulders, head, and eyes to swing easily together. Keep your eyes open and relaxed; make no attempt to focus on anything. Breathe normally as you turn, also in coordination with your swing. Swing easily, gracefully, and pleasurably with your muscles loose.

While doing the exercise, blink somewhat more than usual.

You should swing at a rate of about 16 complete turns a minute, or once every four seconds. Practice the Long Swing for about five minutes before turning out the lights and you should go to bed more relaxed.

TAKE A BATH BEFORE BED

A warm bath before retiring will help increase the circulation to the skin, which should make you sleepy. Prepare your bed before you bathe, perhaps while the tub is filling up. Fill the tub enough to immerse yourself as fully as possible. The water should be warm, never too hot; don't let the water temperature exceed 100° or dip beneath 90°. Body temperature is recommended.

You may improve the soothing qualities of warm water by adding ordinary baking soda. This will make the bath more alkaline and soothe the nerves on the surface of the skin. A few drops of oil of eucalyptus can also be added. A tablespoon of mustard powder or genuine pine needle essence can have a relaxing effect as well. And there's always your favorite balm oil or perfume.

Immerse yourself for about 20 minutes. Close your eyes, dim the bathroom lights or light a candle, and let yourself unwind. Some soft music of your choice will add to the serene atmosphere.

After the bath, dry yourself by patting gently with a fluffy towel. Don't rub—the friction will be stimulating. Then go quietly to bed. And we *do* mean go to bed. We suggested this bath routine to a young woman named Lindsay Garfield and when we asked her how it went she said, "It worked so well I fell asleep in the bath!"

John Lust, author of *The Herb Book,* recommends any of the following formulas to add to the insomniac's bath. In each case add the concoction to your bath water.

1. Steep 2 ounces of balm leaves in a quart of boiling water for 15 minutes.
2. Add 7 ounces of angelica root to 2 quarts of cold water, bring to a boil and steep for 5 minutes.
3. Add 3–4 ounces of valerian root to 1 quart of cold water, let soak for 10–12 hours, and bring to a brief boil.
4. Steep 3–4 ounces of mother-of-thyme in 1 pint of boiling water for 10 minutes.

Footbaths are also highly recommended before bed. Here are two variations:

1. Dip your feet and calves in a deep pot or a tub filled with cold water. Keep them in until the cold becomes uncomfortable or the feet feel warm.
2. Alternate between a hot herbal foot bath and the cold water, beginning with the hot for 1 or 2 minutes, followed by the cold for ½ minute, and alternating in that manner for 15 minutes, ending with cold.

THE WORLD'S OLDEST SLEEP RITUAL

Some psychologists and physicians believe that sex is a valuable pre-sleep ritual; others think that its soporific qualities are exaggerated. Here is what *Vogue* magazine has to say: "Many people believe that orgasm is a highly potent sedative. This may be true for some individuals, but not all. Kinsey in his book *Sexual Behavior of the Human Female* indicated that the period of relaxation after orgasm lasts only a very short time . . . from four to five minutes. What's more, many couples make love during the day and then go to work, drive cars, play tennis, and engage in other activities which would be unsuccessful or downright dangerous if they were very sleepy."

Nonetheless, most people we asked about it say that sex does wonders for their sleep—and for almost everything else.

CHAPTER 9

What to Do in Bed

In the dead of the night I am only one of the dark mil-
lions riding forward in black buses toward the unknown.
F. SCOTT FITZGERALD

Okay, it's time for bed. You've
done everything you can to help yourself get to sleep. Will you
slip quietly into slumber, as nature intended, without having
to resort to any more contrivances, or will you struggle wear-
ily and woozily into another night?

If you have read the material in this book carefully and
given serious thought to your sleep patterns and your life-
style, and if you have followed diligently the recommended
procedures, you might be able to lie down when you get tired
and drift off into a natural sound sleep. If you can't—and on
those inevitable occasions when circumstances prevent you
from being able to—you will need ways of encouraging sleep
at the time you need it most.

There are countless techniques that insomniacs can employ once they are in bed. The one cardinal rule to follow is,
"Trying is prohibited!" The absolutely worst thing you can do
for your sleep is to try too hard to achieve it.

Slumber represents a de-excited state, whereas the act of
trying—even mildly—is an excited state. Effort activates the
brain, and when it is time for sleep, arousal is the exact opposite of what you want. "Sleep, like the Kingdom of Heaven,

is not taken by force," someone once said. So reverse the process: let sleep take *you* by allowing yourself to be a willing prey and a grateful captive.

This chapter offers a variety of techniques for bringing about a receptive state of mind and body. One caveat: Don't become overly dependent on these techniques. Too many writers on sleep—and too many insomniacs—make the mistake of relying exclusively on in-bed methods or gimmicks. Having an effective arsenal of such tools is extremely important, but they are, in a sense, last resorts. If the techniques in this chapter work for you, great. But if your problem is severe or chronic, only the changes in patterns and habits brought about by the previously mentioned approaches will bring lasting results. In-bed practices should be done only when necessary; the goal should always be to fall asleep and stay asleep just by lying down and closing your eyes.

MASSAGE

For relieving muscular tension before sleep, and for just plain feeling good, few procedures can rival a good massage. A massage can greatly improve circulation, particularly in the limbs, and prevent the stiffness and cramping that often interfere with sleep. If you are fortunate enough to have someone with terrific hands who will massage you before sleep, that is probably the best way to take advantage of these benefits. *The Massage Book* by George Downing is an excellent source of instructions on administering massage to another person.

On the assumption that you might not have so cooperative a person around, and because you will want to use massage when it is dark and late and you have only yourself to rely on, we have selected a few relaxing massages that can be self-administered. You might want to precede your massage with a full bath, as prescribed in chapter 8. After patting yourself dry, apply almond or coconut oil to your skin. Do this slowly and in a leisurely manner, without rubbing the skin coarsely.

Here is a good full-body massage you can do sitting up in bed:

Begin with your hands on the top of your head. Press gently but firmly with your palms and fingertips. Move forward slowly, pressing deeply, over the forehead and down over the face (do not lift your hands; slide them along pressing as you go). Linger for a while at whatever points feel particularly tense. Continue down over the throat and chest, stopping at the heart.

Place your hands back on the top of your head. Again press and release, this time going over the back of the head. Come down over the back of the neck, and across the shoulders. Give the neck and shoulder muscles lots of attention, as they tend to gather considerable tension. Then come down over the top of the shoulders and across the chest.

Now take your left hand and grasp the fingertips of the right hand, with your thumb on the underside and your fingers on top. Press and release in the same manner, deeply and firmly but with a gentle motion, moving up the right arm. Come all the way up to the shoulder, then down the chest to the heart. Now go back to the fingertips of the right hand, with your left thumb on top and your fingers on the underside, and repeat the process. Switch arms, massaging your left arm both on top and underneath.

Now place your hands on your belly, middle fingers touching at the navel. Massage your belly and abdomen very gently, then press and release as before, moving up the front of the body to the chest.

Place your hands on your lower back, fingertips touching at the coccyx. Massage up the back and sides, pressing and releasing until you reach as high as you can.

Now for the all-important feet and legs. Grasp the toes of your right foot, right hand on top and left underneath. Massage the toes and feet thoroughly. Now move up the leg, over the ankle and calf, pressing and releasing deeply and thoroughly, but being careful not to cause discomfort or pain. Give your feet and calves as much time as you like, as circulation there is crucial. Come up over the knee and continue in like manner all the way up the thigh. If you care to recline to massage the legs, do so by all means. Lie on your back and bend your knee so you can reach the area you are massaging without having to stretch too far. In some cases, you may not be able to massage from a reclining position until you get to your calf.

Massaging the Upper Body

The upper parts of the body, particularly the face, are often the areas most in need of a bedtime massage. Here are some localized massages for those areas.

Head. Place the index and middle fingers of both hands side by side on top of your head and massage your scalp with deep pressure for about five seconds. Cover your whole scalp in this way. Now move your hands behind your head and place the index and middle fingers of both hands in the slight indentation at the center of the top of your neck, just below the base of the skull. Apply deep pressure for a few seconds, rotating the fingertips in a circular motion. Pause and repeat twice.

Move your hands away from each other along the base of the skull about 1½ to 2 inches (or the width of two fingers), and apply deep pressure there with the index and middle fingers. Move your hands another inch or two and repeat the procedure at the point on the base of the skull adjacent to the ears.

Neck. Place the index and middle fingers of your left hand at the starting point (the top) of the large muscle that runs along the side of the neck from the base of the skull to the shoulder line. Place your right hand in the corresponding position on the other side. Apply deep pressure and massage these points thoroughly for a few seconds. Move your fingers slowly down the muscle lines to your shoulders, applying pressure along the way.

Shoulders. There is a very tender spot slightly to the rear of your shoulder, at the point halfway between the base of the neck and the edge of the shoulder. Find that spot, apply deep pressure with your fingertips, and massage for a few seconds. Repeat a few times on both shoulders—this should go a long way toward removing tension in the shoulders, a key spot.

With the opposite hand, squeeze the outside of your upper arm, then move up toward the shoulder, continuing to squeeze. Apply pressure to the shoulder itself, then move across to the muscle connecting the shoulder and neck. A great deal of tension is stored in that area; it warrants some extra massage time.

Face. This one can be done lying down. Close your eyes. Put both hands lightly over your face. Massage your forehead gently with your fingers in a slow, circular motion. Be very gentle with your face—don't be quite as vigorous as you are with the neck and shoulders. Now slide your hands down a bit and repeat the circular movements, gently, over your eyelids and eye sockets.

Slide your hands down still further, and, with your middle fingers at the corners of your mouth, stroke upward in light, circular movements. Go all the way up to the temples.

Don't forget your scalp. Russian nobles had servants scratch their heads for them when insomnia threatened. The Japanese have a tradition of "skull massage" too. Use light, circular motions to massage the scalp with your fingertips.

Foot Massage

Mrs. Kaufman, the mother of one of the authors, suddenly found herself unable to sleep. The problem lasted for days and had everyone mystified—she had always been healthy and slept like a log from the minute her head hit the pillow. The insomnia lasted for several days, and at the same time she was also beset by a seemingly unrelated problem: her new shoes were too tight and they were hurting her feet because she had

to stand a lot at work. Unlike her sleeplessness, the shoe problem was easy to solve: she started wearing a looser, more
comfortable pair. As a result, her feet felt better during the
day. And, strangely enough, she also slept better at night. It
seems that the constriction of her feet had caused the sort of
irritating, low-grade discomfort that can later interfere with
sleep.

There may be more to that story, and to our feet, than
meets the eye. According to some theories, the various organs,
nerves, and glands in our bodies are connected with certain
reflex areas on the feet. Each specific organ has a known association with a particular point on the sole, toes, ankles, or
heel. For this reason, and because we often spend long hours
standing and walking in shoes of questionable comfort, our
feet might be more important to our sleep—as well as our
overall health—than we imagine. For insomniacs, it is a wise
idea to make sure that the circulation in the feet is unobstructed.

Here is an excellent foot massage for relieving discomfort
and improving circulation:

Sit comfortably with your left leg crossed over the right so
that you can easily grasp the left foot. Using the knuckles of
your right hand, massage the sole of the foot (or you might
use the eraser end of a pencil). Press firmly, moving in small
circles. Cover the entire sole. Go slowly, and don't be squeam-
ish. When you dig into a particularly tender area, you have
probably located crystalline deposits on nerve endings. The
tenderness is an indication that the area needs attention. Dig
in, but be careful not to press hard on ligaments or tendons.

After massaging the entire sole, move to the top of the
foot. Using the tips of your thumbs (not the soft, fleshy pad,
but the tips adjacent to the nail) massage the top of the foot
from the toes to the ankle. As before, massage in a circular
motion. Since the top of the foot exposes more bones and
tendons, you should be gentle but firm.

Along the top of your feet are long tendons that run from

the base of the ankle down to each toe. Press firmly with the tip of your thumb in the valleys between the tendons, and run the thumb down the foot to the toes. Do this in each valley.

Massage the bottom edge of the heel with your fingertips and thumb. Press hard.

Grasp your foot with both hands, pressing your fingertips into the sole. The heels of your hands should meet on top of the foot. Press hard on top and bottom, and slide your hands out to the edges of the foot.

Holding your foot steady with one hand, grasp the big toe with your thumb and forefinger. Pull gently, and shake the toe. Repeat with each toe.

Repeat this entire process on your right foot.

For mechanical assistance in caring for the all-important feet, try the Songrand Footbath, a portable whirlpool bath that churns water around the feet. It is very refreshing, as is Dr. Scholl's Foot Massager, a vibrating pad that you can rest your feet upon while seated for a complete massage.

Take care of your feet, and remember to avoid tight shoes. Or if you must wear them, change into more comfortable ones after work. Better yet, make sure you have the correct size. That often-heard complaint in shoe stores—"But I've always worn a size 6!"—has probably kept many a person awake.

Mechanical Massagers

There are many electronic aids to massage—vibrating and nonvibrating devices of varying sizes and shapes designed to help you access areas of your body you might not be able to reach with your hands. They also enable you to administer greater pressure and stimulation than you can manually. Although you might find the buzzing of an electronic vibrating machine unsettling, the added power might work wonders for tense muscles and spasms.

For insomniacs, the ultimate gadget might be the "Magic Fingers Bed Massager." It attaches to your bed, providing up to 30 minutes of massage at a time. It requires no special tools to set up, and it is said to "convert any bed into a relaxing massager."

ACUPRESSURE

An offshoot of acupuncture and based on the same principles, acupressure—or *shiatsu* in Japanese—has caught on as a cross between its needle-using parent and massage. The technique can be self-administered if you are capable of causing yourself a little pain, for the finger pressure used to stimulate acupuncture points should be firm and vigorous. Using the firm tip of the thumb or forefinger—or a soft-but-strong equivalent such as the eraser end of a pencil—you apply sufficient pressure to cause a sensation that one practitioner describes as "midway between pleasure and pain."

We selected from several sources a few pressure points associated with insomnia. As with acupuncture, stimulating these points is said to correct imbalances in the body. You might perform acupressure on these points while lying in bed. The technique is simple: find the correct point, press firmly with the tip of the thumb or forefinger, and rotate in rapid, counterclockwise circles without moving from the spot (the fingertip should move together with the skin as opposed to rubbing over the surface). The application should last no more than 10 to 15 seconds at first, but may be repeated three or four times. If the point has locations on both sides of the body (e.g., on each arm or leg) perform the technique on each side, one after the other.

We suggest using one of these points at a time so you may evaluate which, if any, work for you. *Note that self-administered acupressure is not advised under the following conditions:* after the third month of pregnancy; on points lying beneath scars, warts, moles, swollen skin, infections, or varicose veins; within four hours of taking medicine or intoxicants; within half an hour of a heavy meal or strenuous physical activity; by sufferers of cancer, cardiac disease, or arthritis.

Point 1. With this one, you might use the thumb and forefinger in a squeezing fashion. Stimulating this point is said to activate the production of serotonin, which we have seen is a neurotransmitter that plays a key role in the sleep mechanism. (See Figure 9-1.)

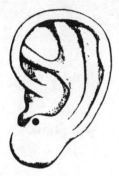

Figure 9-1. Acupressure Point 1.

Point 2. This is located about an inch behind the lobule of the ear. (See Figure 9-2.)

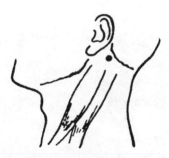

Figure 9-2. Acupressure Point 2.

Point 3. On the crease of the inner wrist, in line with the smallest finger. (See Figure 9-3.)

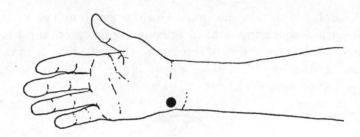

Figure 9-3. Acupressure Point 3.

Point 4. About three inches above the ankle on the inner side of the leg, just behind the tibia. (See Figure 9-4.)

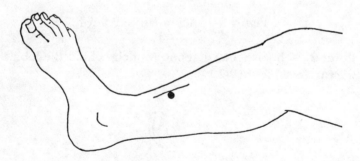

Figure 9-4. Acupressure Point 4.

Point 5. Slightly behind the space between the big toe and the adjacent toe. (See Figure 9-5.)

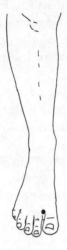

Figure 9-5. Acupressure Point 5.

Point 6. Just below the collarbone (clavicle), in the hollow where the arms join the body. (See Figure 9-6.)

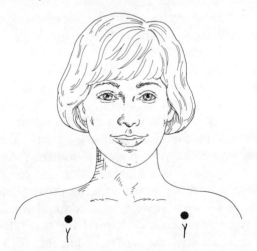

Figure 9-6. Acupressure Point 6.

BREATHING TECHNIQUES

In our own culture and in the East, breathing techniques have been developed for achieving relaxation, improving digestion, and in other ways normalizing the body. Several of these have proven to be significant aids for insomniacs at bedtime.

Deep, abdominal breathing. Few things can calm you down as quickly as a complete deep breath; virtually every expert on stress management advocates the use of this at tense moments.

Most of us breathe in short, shallow breaths, particularly when we are anxious. As a result, stale air is not expelled thoroughly and our tissues are not adequately oxygenated. By learning to breathe with the abdomen instead of just expanding the chest, you can draw more life-enhancing oxygen into your system.

Lying on your back, place your hands on your abdomen, immediately below the navel, with your middle fingertips touching. Breathe through your nose, inhaling slowly, and push your abdomen out as if it were a balloon expanding. Your fingers should separate. As your abdomen expands, your diaphragm will move downward, allowing fresh air to enter the bottom of your lungs.

As the breath continues, expand your chest. More air should now enter, filling the middle part of your lungs. Slightly contracting your abdomen, raise your shoulders and collarbones. This will fill your upper lungs. Hold your breath for a few seconds without straining. Then slowly exhale through your nose, drawing in your abdomen. Your expanded rib cage will return to its normal position and your lungs will empty. Exhaling completely will expel all the stale air.

Experts recommend practicing abdominal breathing a few times a day until it becomes natural for you. The first few sessions might cause slight dizziness, but that is normal. Remember, don't strain in order to retain the breath or go any slower than is comfortable.

Needless to say, deep abdominal breaths can be taken in bed when you are having difficulty calming down. The method is also the preferred way to breathe when practicing other techniques, such as Yoga Mudra in chapter 8 and the two breathing exercises that follow.

The Kelly method.   During sleep, the carbon dioxide level in the blood increases. This, coupled with the fact that carbon dioxide has a natural tranquilizing effect that often brings on drowsiness, led Dr. Charles Kelly to develop a program of controlled breathing that has been found to help people fall asleep. Designed to increase the carbon dioxide level of the blood, these techniques are easy, effective, and free from any possible side effects.

Lie either on your back or on your side, whichever you find more conducive to easy breathing. Make sure your room is dark and well-ventilated. Use a pillow that is just high enough to keep your head straight, or perhaps tilted slightly back. Be sure not to have your head lean forward—when it tilts slightly back the throat and eye muscles relax, and you can breathe more freely.

Close your eyes lightly.

Begin with a few very deep inhalations, filling the lungs and expanding the chest as much as possible. Then exhale fully, drawing in the abdomen to expel as much air as possible. Repeat this three times.

At the end of the third exhalation, when the lungs are as empty as possible, hold your breath for as long as you can. Hold it until the impulse to breathe cannot be resisted easily. Then repeat the three deep breaths, again holding your breath at the end of the third exhalation.

By doing this, you gradually accumulate carbon dioxide in the body. The three deep breaths restore the oxygen content of the blood and remove enough carbon dioxide to allow the breath to be held longer—and, as a result, more carbon dioxide can be produced. The carbon dioxide makes the chemical balance of the blood more acidic, and it slows the activity of the nerves and the brain, preparing them for the onset of natural sleep.

It is important, however, not to take more than three deep breaths in any part of the cycle, to keep the carbon dioxide buildup at just the right level. If you deviate from Kelly's prescription, chances are the carbon dioxide will be eliminated and drowsiness will not come.

When not breathing at the end of the third breath, keep the lungs as empty as possible to prevent the carbon dioxide from being absorbed from the bloodstream by the lungs.

Do not fear that you are being deprived of oxygen. You have more than enough in your bloodstream to nourish your cells, and as soon as you resume normal breathing, your body will balance itself accordingly.

To aid the breath retention, distract your mind from the effort by thinking of a song or a poem you can recite to yourself. Or you may prefer to use one of the other imagination-aids that we will discuss later in this chapter.

Turn your eyes upward during the breathing exercises; it has been found that the position is conducive to sleep.

After perhaps five to eight periods of maximum deep breaths (three per set) and long breath-holding, you will feel a strong desire to breathe normally. You will also feel more relaxed and eager to rest. Quite possibly you will have fallen sleep before you do this five times.

If, after eight repetitions, you still cannot fall asleep, try the following exercise. Do not use it, however, until you have mastered the first.

In this exercise you will again take in as deep a breath as you can, and exhale as much air as you can. As before, do this three times. After the third repetition, however, instead of holding your breath, you will have a period of what Kelly calls "minimum breathing."

"Minimum breathing," says Kelly, "means breathing in and out so slightly that the movement of the air in the nostrils is just perceptible. The minimum breathing must be very shallow and the breaths very short."

Do not fill the lungs with air. Keep the abdomen completely relaxed—don't tense the muscles. Do this until you feel the urge to breathe more deeply. Then start another series of three maximally deep breaths and complete expulsions. After those three, repeat the minimum breathing again.

Continue in this manner for as long as necessary. Be casual about it. You might find your mind drifting so much you forget how many breaths you have taken, or maybe even what you are doing in the first place. That is perfectly fine. Don't struggle to remain alert for the purpose of doing the exercise. The purpose, remember, is to do exactly the opposite—drift into oblivion. Indeed, this technique can often be so effective you will find yourself drifting off during the minimum breathing periods.

Remember to take "rest" periods of normal breathing between repetitions.

Alternate nostril breathing. This is a traditional Yoga practice, customarily done before periods of meditation. It is remarkably calming and is said to restore equilibrium to the nervous system. Do it sitting up in bed comfortably (if you are very sleepy or you are awakened in the night, you might find it more comfortable to do it lying down).

Place the tip of your right thumb against your right nostril. Place the middle and ring fingers against your left nostril. Keep your hand relaxed. Close the right nostril with the thumb and breathe in through the left.

Inhale slowly and easily with the body relaxed. The breath may be slightly deeper than usual, but make no effort to take in an extra quantity of air. Some sources recommend holding the breath for three or four seconds once it is inhaled. We too have found that effective, but when you are drowsy attempting to hold the breath might feel like a strain, in which case don't bother,

Exhale when ready. But exhale through the right nostril, lifting the thumb and closing the left nostril with your other fingers. Exhale slowly and noiselessly, but without straining to go at any particular pace. Follow whatever rhythm is comfortable. Some recommend inhaling and exhaling to a particular count—again, when drowsiness is being encouraged, this might cause strain.

After having exhaled, and perhaps held the breath momentarily, inhale through the right nostril, keeping the left one closed. When you have inhaled and feel the urge to exhale, switch nostrils again, closing the right one this time.

The sequence, then, is as follows: out—in—switch nostrils, out—in—switch nostrils, out—in—switch nostrils, and so on.

You should do this alternate nostril technique for about 5 minutes. After you are accustomed to it, you might increase to 10 minutes. Naturally, if you feel sufficiently drowsy, stop, lie down, and sleep.

If at any point you forget which nostril to close, or whether to inhale or exhale, or if you forget why your fingers are at your nose, then the technique is working. You are likely to be drifting off into sleep.

There are no formal studies of these controlled breathing techniques, but the anecdotal evidence is substantial. In questioning people who have tried many different techniques, we found that many had considerable success with the breathing practices described here, both at bedtime and when awakened during the night. If you do them and still do not fall asleep easily, don't be discouraged. They might work perfectly well at another time.

HYPNOSIS

Discovered in the eighteenth century by the Viennese physician Franz Mesmer, modern hypnosis has had a stormy history. It was not until 1958 that the American Medical Association accepted hypnosis, provided it was done by trained doctors. Now it is widely used by hypnotherapists and psychiatrists to help people overcome specific phobias, fears, and unwanted habits. In qualified therapeutic hands, hypnosis is a far cry from the sideshow novelty that it once was. It has been shown to be an effective way to rid the subconscious mind of destructive thought patterns, one of which might be keeping you awake.

Not everyone can be hypnotized; it requires a certain amount of faith in the hypnotist and the determination to do what the hypnotist suggests. Even at that, some subjects are more susceptible than others. If you would like to try hypnotherapy, keep in mind the following: Hypnosis has been helpful in countering the fear of not being able to fall asleep, which can often be self-fulfilling. Hypnosis has also been used to foster the will to sleep and to restore confidence to an insomniac who has come to wonder if sleep will ever be possible again. It has also been effective in countering the reverse apprehension, the subconscious fear of losing control or of being vulnerable to harm, which some believe is the root cause of many insomnias.

However, to a certain degree hypnosis does involve a surrender of willpower. There is a chance you will become dependent on the hypnotist, or on the subterfuge of suggestion—which some argue is unnatural—and be unable to fall asleep any other way. These are matters to discuss with a hypnotherapist in advance.

One person we interviewed, a computer programmer named Shirley Todd, swore by hypnosis. "I tried all sorts of things to help me sleep," she said. "Finally I went to a doctor who recommended a hypnotherapist. At first, I was afraid of putting myself in the hands of a stranger. But he quickly won my confidence. He was certain he could put me to sleep. And he did. Right in his office. He shut the lights and told me to relax. I can't recall his exact words, but he told me, essentially, that I was getting tired—he used words like heavy, floating, drifting, and so on. At first I giggled, but after a while I was dozing off. Next thing I knew, he was waking me up from a deep nap. He gave me a tape to play before bed, with basically the same sort of suggestions on it. It works like a charm."

Not all hypnotists provide tapes, of course, although they are becoming more and more common. Most often, the hypnotist will induce the trancelike state deemed necessary for implanting the suggestion in his office. Once having been made, the suggestion should then trigger the conditioned reaction at the appropriate time—presumably, when it's time to go to sleep.

Many nonsleepers try to employ the do-it-yourself variety, known as *self-hypnosis* or *autosuggestion*. One of the most famous examples of this appears in the writings of the French scientist Emile Coué, who created a rage in the 1920s when he came up with the self-suggestion refrain, "Day by day, in every way, I grow better and better."

Coué wrote: "Every night when you have comfortably settled yourself in bed, you will repeat (not gobble), 'I am going to sleep, I am going to sleep,' in a quiet, placid, even voice, avoiding of course the slightest mental effort to obtain the result. The soporific effect of this droning repetition soon makes itself felt, whereas, if one actually tries to sleep, the spirit of wakefulness is kept alive by the negative idea, according to the law of converted effort."

Coué's basic method is used—in a thousand variations—by the modern form of autosuggestion, the *affirmation*. To be effective, affirmations should always be framed in a permissive, positive tone, using such words as "I can," "I will," or "I am going to." So statements such as "I can fall sleep easily and not wake up until I am refreshed" are preferred over negatively phrased suggestions such as "I am not going to stay awake" or "I won't have insomnia any longer." Also, a suggestion is not the same as a command—don't issue orders to yourself (as in, "Go to sleep!") as though you could be forced to obey.

Experts on autosuggestion caution that instant results should not be expected because it takes time for the suggestions to be implanted in the subconscious. Since confidence is an absolute must, self-hypnotists are advised not to set themselves up for a fall by attempting big objectives at the beginning. Start simple and work your way up.

In a sense, self-suggestion is something we all do much of the time. We are always telling ourselves that we are going to do something, or change something, or turn over a new leaf. And those injunctions are often countered by contradictory voices from our subconscious that nullify our intentions by whispering "You can't . . ." or "You'll never . . ." like some mean-spirited nag. Autosuggestion is a way of affirming the positive voices and canceling the negative ones.

The potential problem with self-hypnosis and sleep is that although the willpower you induce through suggestion might increase your determination, it could also keep you awake by inducing that archenemy of sleep: trying.

Here is a form of self-hypnosis supplied by one hypno therapist we spoke with:

"Lie on your back in bed, with your arms at your sides and your hands open. The room should be dark and quiet. Breathe deeply for two minutes, mentally saying to yourself, 'I will soon be fast asleep.' Then concentrate on the following suggestions. Repeat them for about five minutes: 'I am very comfortable, so very comfortable. My arms are heavy. My feet are heavy. My eyes are heavy. Everything is slowing down. I am floating and drifting. I want to fall asleep. I am beginning to fall asleep.' Repeat these, or words like them, and soon the feelings they describe will be felt, and you should fall asleep."

The hypnotist said that there are countless variations on this theme, including repeating the suggestions to the rhythm of deep breathing and doing them along with techniques for muscle relaxation such as the Jacobson method.

We cannot vouch for any particular self-hypnotic technique, although it is certainly plausible that any of them can help an insomniac get to sleep. Certainly, our minds are capable of exerting their wills over our bodies, and hypnosis is a proven treatment for many maladies. However, some sleep experts question whether the sleep induced by hypnosis is natural sleep and whether the suggestions ever become anything more than sophisticated self-deception.

"In hypnosis," says Dr. Peter Steincrohn, an expert on relaxation, "the typical brain-wave changes observed during normal sleep do not occur, the knee-jerk reflex still operates, and the usual falls in blood pressure and pulse rate do not take place." Says French physician Paul Chauchard, director of the Ecole des Hautes Etudes in Paris: "Hypnotists work by paralyzing the part of the nerve center (in the brain) that controls sleep, but their method does not promote normal sleep. The sensitive nerve mechanisms are merely thrown out of action by upsetting their inner metabolism. This does not bring true repose."

If you choose to try hypnosis, remember it does not work for everyone. You should consult with an experienced clinical hypnotist to see if you are a likely candidate. Your local medical society, the psychiatry department of your local hospital, or the psychology department of your local university should be able to recommend reliable therapists who use hypnosis.

BEDTIME RELAXATION TECHNIQUES

The literature on sleep contains a great number of relaxation exercises designed to reduce tension at bedtime. Many of these are variations on the Corpse Pose, described in our section on Yoga, where you will each part of your body to relax progressively. Others are variations on Jacobson's Progressive Relaxation technique (which can be done in bed even though it was presented in an earlier chapter). We reviewed the available procedures and here offer those that are easy to perform and have a relatively immediate impact on muscular tension.

We recommend first that you give nature a chance on its own. When you turn off the lights and lie down, just lie there.

Be easy, don't do anything in particular, mentally or physically, and see what happens. If, after 5 to 10 minutes, the tension in your muscles does not diminish, or gets worse, or your mind is still racing, then begin using these techniques.

When you use these techniques (or any others for that matter), be extremely casual. Do not attempt to concentrate. If your mind drifts, let it go—it might be going to sleep. If you forget the sequence of exercises, or if you forget where you were because your mind wandered, don't get upset. Just proceed, and stop whenever you start drifting toward sleep.

The Steincrohn method. Physician Peter Steincrohn recommends the following procedure for in-bed relaxation:

Lying on your back in a dark, quiet room, clench your right fist tightly and raise it off the bed with all your muscles tensed. Hold for about a minute. Then let the arm go limp and drop it to the bed. After a few seconds, repeat the procedure with the left arm and fist. Then do it again, one arm at a time, only this time let the tension decrease *gradually* until the arm is completely limp.

Next, push both toes downward as far as they will go. Hold for a minute. Then suddenly stop the tension. Repeat, but this time let the tension decrease very gradually.

Then, expand your chest by breathing in more deeply than usual. Hold your breath for a few seconds. Then let your chest go suddenly limp. Again, repeat the procedure, relaxing the muscles gradually.

Now the forehead and face. Raise your eyebrows so your forehead moves up. Then relax it. Then lower the forehead in a frown and relax it. Repeat with gradual relaxing.

Next, the eyes. Look as far as you can toward your right ear (remember your eyes are closed) and hold for 10 or 20 seconds. Relax, wait a moment, and look toward your left ear. Again hold, then relax. Next, look up toward your hairline, hold, then relax. Finally, look toward your chin, hold, and relax. As before, repeat each step, relaxing your muscles more gradually.

The last area is the speech area. Count out loud to 10. Notice the tension produced in the throat, lips, tongue, and face. Now relax all those muscles. Repeat the count, using less and less muscular effort, counting softer and softer. Then do it again, trying not to use the speech muscles at all.

If you practice this series of exercises—essentially, tensing and relaxing—after a while you should be able to quickly trigger relaxation for the full range of muscles.

The Pai method.   Dr. N. M. Pai, a staunch opponent of the use of sleeping pills long before it became fashionable to speak out on the matter, advocates what he calls the "Tenlax" method:

Lie comfortably on your back in a quiet, dark room, eyes closed. Tense your muscles by stretching your legs, and pointing your toes away from you. Pressing the back downward, hold your legs in as tense a position as possible for as long as you can. Let go suddenly. After a moment, repeat the procedure. Do this six times.

Now tense the muscles of your arms, clenching the fists as tightly as you can. Hold for as long as it is not unbearable. Let go suddenly. Repeat this six times.

Eyes still closed, focus as though you were looking at the end of your nose. Relax. Then focus on your hairline. And relax.

Dr. Pai believes that this series of maneuvers should be enough to lower anxiety in most people. For those who have been chronically sleep-deprived, especially if they have been taking pills for it, Dr. Pai recommends the following:

In the same setting and position, close off one nostril and exhale through the other. Then inhale. Switch nostrils, exhale and inhale, and switch again, alternately.

While doing this, tense your leg muscles, pointing your toes, and lifting the legs slightly. Hold the legs in that manner for as long as you can. Then let go, dropping the legs.

Now discontinue the alternate breathing and breathe normally. Clench your fists, hold for 20 seconds, and let go. Wait half a minute. Then raise your head and shoulders off your bed and hold for 20 seconds. Let go.

Back to the legs. Stretch your right leg, pointing the toes. Tense the whole leg and hold it off the bed for 15 seconds. And let go. Now switch your legs and repeat the entire procedure. Continue to do this, alternating legs, a total of four times.

Now to the arms. Clench your fists. Bend your elbows completely, with the arm muscles tense, and hold for as long as you can while simultaneously holding your breath. And let go. Take a deep breath and relax completely, turning your eyes upward.

Dr. Pai says that many of his patients sleep soundly after a few lessons. While doing any of Dr. Pai's exercises, stop as soon as you feel you are near falling asleep.

A technique from the Yoga tradition. Lying in bed on your back, raise your right arm above your head so that it is in a straight line with your body. Stretch your right side from toes to fingers. Notice the feeling of tension, while reaching as far as you can. Then release. After a moment, repeat the process on your left side.

Now stretch the nape of your neck and pull in your chin. Let go.

Now put your palms on top of your head and pull backward for half a minute.

Open your mouth as wide as you can, then release. Repeat three or four times.

Now hold your tongue against the side of your cheek for ten seconds. And release.

Bug your eyes out for ten seconds. And relax.

Now massage each finger and thumb, shake your hands up and down and sideways. Bend your arm over your chest, clenching your fist. Tense the whole arm, then relax. Repeat three or four times, alternating arms.

Pulling your toes toward you, press your legs against each other hard. Hold for a minute or more, then relax. Repeat until you notice the absence of tension in your legs.

Now expand your chest as much as possible, hold for a few seconds, and let go, exhaling slowly. Repeat until you feel relaxed in the chest muscles. Then exhale, pulling in your stomach as far as possible. Hold a few seconds and let go. Repeat several times.

Now yawn and go to sleep.

The Tongue-in-Cheek method. Dr. Steincrohn has observed that his insomniac patients often pressed their tongues hard against the roofs of their mouths or against the back ridge of their upper teeth. He suggests a way to relax the tense muscles around the jaw:

Let your tongue relax by pulling it away from the roof of your mouth or the back of your teeth, and gently slide it between your teeth, against the inner cheeks. Hold it there for a few minutes. It should help you relax.

Dr. Steincrohn claims that this simple method is the most effective device he knows for relieving tension-related insomnia.

THE EYES HAVE IT

On the battlefields of World War I, a fortuitous discovery was made by the famous neurologist Dr. Foster Kennedy. As he watched the British army retreat, Dr. Kennedy saw soldiers so exhausted that they fell on the ground where they were and plunged into a sleep as deep as a coma. They didn't even wake up when the doctor raised their eyelids with his fingers.

While raising those eyelids, Dr. Kennedy noticed that, invariably, the pupils of the soldiers' eyes were rolled upward in their sockets. "After that," Dr. Kennedy wrote, "when I had trouble sleeping, I would practice rolling up my eyeballs into this position, and I found that in a few seconds I would begin to yawn and feel sleepy. It was an automatic reflex over which I had no control."

Since then, Dr. Kennedy's observation has been confirmed. Experiments have shown that we always fall asleep with our eyes in an upward position.

Whatever the explanation (some have suggested fatigue of the eye muscles, for example), keeping the eyes directed upward by looking over the head—figuratively speaking, since your eyes should be closed—will often help bring on sleep. You might even start the process with your eyes open: Stare at a spot above your head so that your eyes are required to rise to the top of the sockets. Open and close the eyes in this position a few times, then keep them closed for sleep.

Here is another technique for the eyes, advocated by Aldous Huxley in his *The Art of Seeing:* Warm your hands by rubbing them briskly together. Now place the palms lightly over your eyes with the sides of your hands against the sides of your nose. Don't exert pressure on your eyeballs, but keep all light from entering your eyes. A minute or two of this warming, soothing influence on the eyes can be remarkably calming.

WHAT TO DO ABOUT LEG JITTERS

In chapter 4 we described an illness known as *nocturnal myoclonus.* Known colloquially as *leg jitters,* or *restless legs,* this condition prevents the victim from keeping his or her legs still while lying down to sleep. The condition, which is often associated with similar leg-jerking during wakefulness, is quite common, and it occurs on and off for many insomniacs.

The earliest known description of myoclonus was made back in 1695 by the great clinical neurologist Dr. Thomas Willis: "Wherefore to some, when being a Bed they betake themselves to sleep, presently in the Arms and Leggs, Leapings and Contractions of the Tendons, and so great a Restlessness and Tossings of their Members ensue, that the diseased are no more able to sleep, than if they were in a Place of the greatest Torture."

Modern sufferers of leg jitters have described the sensations involved in various ways—as creeping, pulling, or stretching inside the leg itself. In some cases the jerking, which has been described as "diabolical," might last for several hours, during which time it is impossible to fall asleep.

The exact cause of restless legs is uncertain, although there are some indications that it might be associated with a vitamin deficiency or anemia. Taking iron pills is said to help, especially during the last third of pregnancy when as many as 10 percent of women report having some experience of restless legs. Regular large doses of ascorbic acid (vitamin C) can also be beneficial. Other treatments include aspirin and vasodilator drugs such as Roniacal. Mild cases might be alleviated with exercise.

Dr. Steincrohn, whom we have quoted several times, claims that an effective treatment for leg jitters is to soak in a hot bath and then do 10 deep knee-bends.

If you have this condition recurrently, and if none of the above suggestions works, see your doctor or go to the nearest sleep clinic.

POINT YOUR HEAD IN THE RIGHT DIRECTION

Carl Reichenbach, the inventor of paraffin, used to say that in cases of insomnia the person should simply turn around and sleep with his head at the foot of the bed.

We don't know if Reichenbach's method worked or not, but if the insomniac happened to be pointing in the wrong direction it just might have. Many different folk stories allude to the effects of pointing your head in a certain direction. Charles Dickens, for example, would not go anywhere without a compass. He insisted on sleeping with his head pointed north and would move the furniture in his room over the protests of innkeepers.

Dickens might have been on to something more than superstition. Studies of men in the polar regions have shown that sleep is more difficult there. Despite the heavy work they were doing, few of the men studied at the poles had any Stage IV sleep. And when they returned to their homelands, it took a full year to reestablish their previous sleep patterns. According to a government study, the reason for this aberration was the magnetic field at the pole.

Other research has demonstrated the effects of magnetic fields. A Canadian study, for example, showed that patients with mental disorders had periods of extreme mobility and increased disorientation whenever there were sunspots or large magnetic changes caused by the weather.

The question is, if direction matters, which is the right direction? Dickens insisted it was the north, as do many others. However, according to certain Indian texts, north is the *least* desirable direction in which to point, east being the preferred orientation.

Why not vary directions every few nights to see if any one has an effect on your sleep? You might find, as many have, that direction makes a difference.

THE BEST POSITION TO SLEEP IN

An old Islamic proverb states that only kings may sleep on the right side, the left side is for wise men, saints may sleep on their backs, and it's the devil's privilege to sleep on his stomach.

In our own culture, psychologists have studied our favorite sleeping postures. Dr. Samuel Dunkell, author of *The Sleep Position: The Night Language of the Body*, claims that "a preferrred sleeping position is stubbornly clung to because it expresses how we feel about the world." Dunkell describes an amazing and amusing range of positions with clever names such as "flamingo," "monkey," "cyclops," "sphinx," "chain gang," and "swastika." He says, for example, that sleeping flat on the back in what he calls the royal posture, expresses openness and unusual confidence.

Whatever the subconscious reasons, your position in bed can make a difference in how well you sleep. For one thing, faulty posture can cut off the circulation to various parts of the body, which might either awaken you or make your sleep inefficient. It might even create physical problems, to which you might ascribe the wrong cause. J. I. Rodale, founder of *Prevention* magazine, says he once eliminated a persistent neuritis when he realized that he laid his head on his arm during sleep. The pressure was pinching his nerves.

Most experts counsel against sleeping on your stomach—it is not good for the neck muscles, or for breathing. Lying on the back is not the top choice, but is considered superior to lying on your stomach. If you lie on your back, you might try placing a pillow or two under your knees (there are wedge-shaped pillows made specifically for this purpose). Some people advocate the use of bed blocks, or decks—wooden or plastic wedges that raise the mattress at the foot of the bed (or at the head of the bed, for reading). Said to aid circulation, these devices have the added advantage of discouraging you from lying on your stomach. Several manufacturers produce beds that can be adjusted to raise the back and provide leg support.

The ideal position for sleeping is shown in Figure 9-7. In this position, the spine is in a straight line; the knees and elbows are relaxed, with the limbs free of the body; the body is anchored by the bones, not by the pull of muscles; shoulders and hips are firmly set. The hands and feet can be moved to positions that are comfortable for your particular build. A thin pillow may be placed under the uppermost knee, if you like. This position gives you lots of freedom for the 20 to 35 position changes we each make during the night.

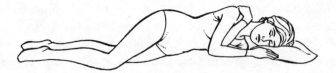

Figure 9-7. The ideal sleeping position.

Remember, although this might be the ideal sleep position and has the endorsement of sleep experts and posture specialists, if you have been accustomed to a different position for a long time it may take a while to readjust. Also, you will probably find yourself falling back on your old postures during the night. Take your time retraining yourself.

"I had always slept on my stomach," said insomniac Charlie Clarke, "and I had neck problems all my life. When I finally connected the two, I tried to sleep on my side. It was virtually impossible at first. Then I decided to go about it systematically. I started out by lying on my side, and I stayed in that position until I couldn't stand it any longer, and I tried to extend the time a little bit each night. It took weeks before I could fall asleep in that position, but finally I did. When I caught myself lying on my stomach I turned over on my side. Gradually, I kicked the habit of sleeping on my stomach, and both my neck and my sleep improved."

Mark Twain wrote characteristically witty advice about sleep positions: "If you can't sleep, try lying on the end of the bed—then you might drop off."

USE YOUR IMAGINATION

How do people go to sleep? I'm afraid I've lost the knack. I might try busting myself smartly over the temple with the nightlight. I might repeat to myself, slowly and soothingly, a list of quotations beautiful from minds profound; if I can remember any of the damn things.

CHARACTER IN A DOROTHY PARKER STORY

A good many people advocate the use of mind games, such as repeating "a list of quotations beautiful from minds profound," to coax sleep. Others feel that such exercises only keep the mind active and are therefore antagonistic to sleep. In this view, you might get so caught up in a mind game that you struggle to keep awake just to complete it, or to get to the bottom of some perplexing puzzle you have contrived.

That being said, mind games have also been found useful if not for inducing sleep then at least for keeping the mind on relatively cheerful distractions when it might otherwise get bogged down in worries, especially worries over losing sleep. "The chief virtue of brain games," writes Hillary Rubenstein, author of the delightful *Insomniacs of the World, Goodnight*, "is that they keep the mind occupied in a psychologically harmless way. . . . I find that a session of compiling crossword clues, for instance, makes me much less of a tosser and turner than worrying about work, and sooner or later, my mind has had enough of its early morning exercise and I drop off once again."

There is, of course, an infinite variety of things to imagine, scenes to create, games to play, puzzles to solve, and fantasies to indulge in. Some people find it profoundly relaxing to imagine being on some tropical island swimming, or fishing, or to imagine any other idyllic scene that revives a good memory or gives them a worthwhile expectation. Visualizing a favorite person, recalling times of great joy or love—or projecting some anticipated scene of that nature—are also favorites.

One sound sleeper, sportswriter Clark Hanson, told us his secret: "As soon as I close my eyes, I imagine a baseball scene. It is usually the last inning of the last game of the World Series. It's two out, the score is tied, and the bases are loaded. I am either the centerfielder or the relief pitcher just brought in from the bullpen. If I'm in center field, the batter hits a tremendous fly ball that I overhaul by leaping to the top of a ten-foot fence, catching it just before the ball reaches the stands. If I'm the relief pitcher, I strike the batter out. Then, after leaving the field to the appreciative roar of the crowd, I lead off the bottom of the ninth with a game-winning home run. I usually fall asleep before I get to the locker room for the champagne party."

Mr. Hanson says he has been falling asleep to that tune ever since he was 10 years old.

Some people need a more protective fantasy to overcome the fears of the night. One scientist, for example, arranges around the edge of her bed a squadron of protective jungle beasts, all on guard, facing outward, keeping a watchful eye on the door to her room. Others perform practices that border on self-hypnosis, such as imagining that their hands, arms, legs, and feet are slowly turning to lead.

Lewis Carroll used to invent mathematical games to counter his insomnia. In 1888 he published a book called *Curiosa Mathematica,* which contained a section on "Pillow Problems."

Spelling words backwards; naming towns, countries, baseball players, authors, in alphabetical order; plotting a trip across the country to see if you know the map; naming the capital of every state; naming every city (country, author, movie star, etc.) that begins with the letter q, z, or y—all these have been suggested. The possibilities are endless, of course, and there is always the perennial counting sheep.

You might try a technique that has had some clinical success. It was developed by Anees A. Sheikh, a psychology professor at Marquette University. First, you are asked to recall a past occasion when you were fatigued but had to fend off sleep because of external demands—studying for an exam, working late, a long motor trip, or a deadline. Then, you concentrate on the mental image of that situation. You should quickly become drowsy. And then you are told to disregard the demand that forced you to stay awake in the original instance. In this way, you reverse the results and fall asleep instead of remaining awake as you did in the actual situation.

Dr. Sheikh advises insomniacs to experiment with different images and settle on one that works. It must be a real situation, not a hypothetical one.

Finally, here is a visualization exercise designed by the renowned hypnotherapist Dr. Ernest Rossi. Dr. Rossi suggests that you turn your attention to the "comfort zones" in your body. That is, tune in to the places in your body that feel most comfortable, whether your stomach, your arms, your legs, or wherever. Now, put your attention on that feeling of comfort and let it deepen and spread from one of those places throughout your entire body.

Then ask yourself, "What color is the comfort?" When a color comes to your mind's eye associated with the feeling of comfort, visualize the color spreading like a river of light throughout your body. Then imagine your favorite music—a peaceful melody associated with tranquility—and listen to it with your mind's ear.

Finally, become aware of a favorite image, perhaps a scene from nature—the sky or ocean, for example—or the face of someone you love, or a beautiful painting. Let your attention drift to that image, and then drift off to sleep.

Those who would rather have someone else lead the way to slumber might consider purchasing an audio cassette and listening to it in bed. We have written and narrated a one-hour tape—*The Audio Guide to Natural Sleep* (Audio Renaissance Tapes)—that combines practical information with soothing music and guided relaxation and visualization procedures. Other tapes on sleep include *How to Fall Asleep and Stay Asleep*, by Drs. Art Ulene and Michael Stevenson, and the following, which were recommended by the Bodhi Tree bookstore in Los Angeles: *Easing into Sleep* by Emmett Miller; *Reduced Sleep/Improved Sleep* by Jach Pursel; and *Sound Sleep* by Steven Halpern. The Halpern tape features music and subliminal suggestion.

WHAT TO DO ABOUT SNORING

Reportedly, one of every eight Americans snores. That means that on any given night over 30 million snorers are competing with owls and other night creatures, sending out a dissonant drone that is probably keeping a large number of would-be sleepers awake. Although snoring is the subject of a great many jokes, it is no laughing matter to the person who sleeps in the same room with a snorer. Snoring has been the cause of torment in honeymoon suites, college dormitories, and army barracks throughout the world. And the sad thing about it is: it hurts only those who hear it, not those who do it.

What is snoring? Most descriptions say that it is caused by air going past the soft palate and the uvula, the soft piece of tissue that hangs down the back of the throat. Various experts attribute snoring to nasal obstructions caused by enlarged adenoids or tonsils, deviated nasal septums, polyps, allergies, or excessive smoking and drinking. Another explanation is that when lying on the back (the position in which most snoring occurs) the back of the person's tongue might fall against the throat walls, forming a kind of mechanical constriction that causes the tongue and throat tissues to vibrate.

What can you do about an inveterate snorer besides sleeping in a separate room or wearing earplugs? There is a wide range of techniques ranging from the practical to the ludicrous. Here are some that lean toward the former:

Wake up the snorer each time he or she begins to snore. This takes persistence and dedication.

Have the snorer adjust his or her sleeping position so as to discourage breathing through the mouth. For example, have him sleep on his side with his forearm under his chin to keep the mouth closed; or, have him cup a hand under his chin. If the snorer must sleep on her back, place a small pillow under the nape of her neck or place a small pillow under her chin, held in place by an elastic strap to keep the mouth closed.

Prevent turning over onto the back by placing pillows in the way or attaching an obstruction to the snorer's pajamas. (During the Revolutionary War, soldiers sewed a pocket on the back of their nightclothes and inserted a ball or block of wood to discourage turning over onto the back.)

Use a humidifier to increase the humidity in the room. Membranes swollen from too much dryness can cause snoring.

Suggest that snorers reduce their intake of cheese, milk, and bread, since these foods can cause a buildup of mucus that can obstruct breathing.

Is your snorer overweight? Obese persons are more prone to snoring. It's yet another reason, besides good health, to lose weight.

A smart gift idea for the snorer nearest your heart is the Snore Pillow. Said to be used in hospitals and endorsed by Dr. Steven H. Feinsilver, director of the Sleep Disorders Center at the State University of New York, the pillow is constructed to "prevent snoring by providing proper support of the head from any sleeping position." It's available through the mail from Ryans, 23010 Lake Forest Dr., Ste. D321, Laguna Hills, CA 92653; (800) 950-5432.

A habitual snorer should see an ear, nose, and throat specialist. If some obstruction in the nose is the cause of the snoring it can be cured by medical treatment—nose drops, sprays, or antihistamines—or by surgery designed to open up the passages for free breathing.

WHY NOT GET UP AND DO SOMETHING?

Leave your bed upon the first desertion of sleep; it being ill for the eyes to read lying, and worse for the mind to be idle; since the head during laziness is commonly a cage for unclean thoughts.

FRANCIS OSBORN, *English writer*

Some experts believe that insomniacs should remain in bed no matter what, because the body benefits from the rest even if sleep doesn't come. Others believe that a bed is for sleeping in and the more you limit its function to just that the better you will sleep when you are in it.

Like the sleep experts, insomniacs are divided between those who stay in bed and those who get up. In the former category are many who *feel* like getting up but whose ravaged bodies simply won't cooperate. Among those who prefer to get out of bed are many who simply do not like to waste time. Since lost time is the one thing that insomniacs can't make up, they jump out of bed the minute they realize that trying to fall asleep would be futile. They would agree with sleep researcher Joseph Mendels, who said, "The most important thing in bed is not to toss and turn. If you are restless, sit up, turn the lights on, and read for a while, or get up and do something else. Tossing and turning tends to aggravate the cycles of not sleeping—you become more tense and make the situation worse."

If you do get out of bed, you will be in good company, historically speaking. Alexandre Dumas, author of *The Three Musketeers*, was a notorious insomniac who tried all manner of cures until a famous doctor told him to get out of bed when he couldn't sleep. Dumas took to wandering the streets of town watching the sunrise from a hill, or strolling along a riverbank—pre-dawn excursions that inspired some lovely prose. Once his anxiety was relieved, Dumas was able to sleep soundly.

Robert Louis Stevenson was also fond of nighttime expeditions. "I have not often enjoyed a more serene possession of myself, nor felt more independent of material aids," said the author of *Treasure Island* and *The Strange Case of Dr. Jekyll and Mr. Hyde*. "We have a moment to look upon the stars. And there is a special pleasure for some minds in the reflection that we share the impulse with all outdoor creatures in our neighborhood, that we have escaped out of the Bastille of civilisation, and are become, for the time being, a mere kindly animal and a sheep of Nature's flock."

Remember when you were a child and your parents made you go to sleep? Remember how you protested? Remember how little it bothered you then to be unable to fall asleep, or to awaken early? You talked to your toys, you imagined marvelous adventures, you sorted out your baseball cards or tidied up your dollhouse. You enjoyed a rare moment of privacy. Sleep was a nuisance then. What happened? It might not be a bad idea to try to recapture the childlike happiness of the waking state so you can make better use of the fact that you can't sleep. You may even come to count it as a blessing in disguise.

Twentieth-century insomniacs have an edge on Dumas and Stevenson: you can do pretty much anything at night that you can do during the day. You need not have a great imagination to occupy yourself if you are reasonably alert. You may even come up with creative ideas that might not come during the hustle-bustle of the day. How about a trip outdoors? The air is fresher and the streets are quieter at night than they are when the rest of the world is up and about. Of course, if you live in a city, the "outdoor creatures in our neighborhood" may be somewhat unsavory, so you might not want to go out alone. How about forming an insomniac's club? There are precedents for such organizations. One group used to pass the night on "insomniac bicycle tours" of Manhattan.

So, if you can't lick insomnia, try joining it. "It is at night," wrote American author Brian Aldiss, "that the mind is most clear, that we are most able to hold all our life in the palm of our skull."

BOOTZIN'S STIMULUS CONTROL THERAPY

On the theory that remaining in bed while sleepless can reinforce insomnia, psychologist Richard R. Bootzin of Northwestern University devised a simple behavioral therapy that many sleep researchers consider the most important treatment innovation in the field. Bootzin's method is a way of overcoming what he calls the "misuse of bed."

The technique is designed to help insomniacs break their negative conditioning regarding sleep—what Dr. Michael Stevenson, director of the North Valley Sleep Disorders Center in Mission Hills, California, calls "the reflexive, phobic reaction to the bedroom." Apparently, many people who have had bouts of insomnia come to hate the night because they dread not being able to sleep. Then, of course, they *can't* sleep because their dread makes them so tense. Somewhere along the line, the pillow, the bed, the lamp, and the rest of the bedroom environment become cues, not for drowsiness, but for increased alertness and arousal. And so the sufferer tosses and turns.

Dr. Bootzin's regimen is intended to recondition the insomniac to bedtime conditions that have become signals for tension and wakefulness. In other words, to strengthen the association between the bed and natural sleep. Here are the basic guidelines, which can be followed on your own:

Go to bed only when you are tired, no matter how unreasonable the hour.

If sleep does not come in 10 minutes from the time you close your eyes, get out of bed. In fact, get out of the bedroom entirely. The bed must come to be viewed as a place to sleep, not to worry about problems, or to read, watch television, eat, or whatever. Most therapists make one exception to this rule: sex.

During this period away from the bedroom, engage yourself in activities that are relatively nonstimulating. Repetitive tasks such as needlepoint, solitaire, or foreign language practice are recommended. If you do something rewarding or pleasurable, it might reinforce the habit of awakening.

Return to the bedroom only when you think you can fall asleep.

If you do not fall asleep within 10 minutes, once again get out of the room.

Continue this pattern of going to bed and getting up until you fall asleep, never remaining in bed longer than 10 minutes.

If at any time you awaken, give yourself the same 10 minutes to fall back to sleep, and get up if sleep doesn't come.

Use an alarm clock to wake you at the same time every morning, including weekends. Don't oversleep, even if you hadn't fallen asleep until a few minutes before the alarm went off.

Don't nap during the day.

It might require some fortitude to get through the first few days of reconditioning. The experts say it is worth it. Peter Hauri of the Mayo Clinic describes a typical patient: "On the first night of this treatment, the patient usually won't sleep at all; he'll feel miserable the whole day after. But the following night, being tired, he'll get off to sleep somewhere about 3:00 or 4:00 in the morning. The night after that he stays awake for something like three hours. The next night it might be two. And then the individual gets happy, because he sees that it's going to work. Within about two to three weeks, many chronic insomniacs can be retrained in this way so that they can just hit the pillow and fall asleep."

Dr. Bootzin's basic procedure has been used on hundreds of patients and has been generally lauded by the specialists. A 1987 study reported in the journal *Sleep* took 35 patients with a mean history of 15.4 years of insomnia and treated them by restricting their time in bed and promising an extended time in bed if their sleep efficiency improved. At the end of eight weeks, the patients experienced an increase in total sleep time and improvements in sleep latency (the amount of time it takes to fall asleep) and sleep efficiency. Follow-up reports indicated that the improvement remained significant for most patients for several months after treatment. The researchers' conclusion: "Although compliance with the restricted schedule is difficult for some patients, sleep restriction therapy is an effective treatment for common forms of chronic insomnia."

Our research has shown that insomniacs should feel encouraged by recent trends. The growing number of sleep disorder centers bodes well for those with serious, chronic difficulties that require expert medical help. Furthermore, the expansion of knowledge generated by these centers is already trickling down to local doctors' offices and "second tier" diagnostic clinics, bringing benefits to insomniacs with mild or intermittent problems.

In general, the treatment of insomnia—traditionally a hit-and-miss proposition—is on the way to becoming more precise and more natural. Perhaps the most heartening development is that the cavalier dispensing of sleeping pills and the voluntary purchase of over-the-counter sedatives by the public have decreased markedly. Despite the medical community's long-standing history of seeking "magic bullets" to treat symptoms, and the marketing sophistication of the pharmaceutical industry, the truth about sleep drugs has changed the way doctors and patients deal with insomnia. Remedies and treatment regimens that once would have been dismissed as quackery are now gaining acceptance. This reflects another encouraging sign: the growing recognition that sleep problems must be viewed in a holistic context, taking into account the sufferer's mind, body, spirit, and environment.

At the same time, we remain somewhat uneasy about what might be excessive reliance on expensive technology. Our habit of looking for a technological fix has, in the past, led to unwanted and costly side effects. In the case of insomnia, the use of high-tech gadgetry might be out of proportion to the nature of the problem. Insomnia is hardly a life-threatening disease; it strikes us as a mistake for the average insomniac to depend on technology. Procedures that build self-reliance would be more fruitful.

If we might conclude with a wish for the future, it would be for more systematic research done on natural remedies for sleep disorders. Although the acceptance of nondrug treatments has increased significantly, there remains a dearth of formal studies. It is astonishing and disturbing to note the degree to which nutrition, exercise, relaxation procedures, herbs, and other simple, self-administered methods are ignored by researchers. We need more official data to confirm or refute the informal experiments conducted by insomniacs and open-minded physicians.

Finally, we must remember that sleep should be the most natural of events; failure to fall asleep or remain asleep represents a breakdown of the fundamental relationship between an individual and the natural rhythms of life. Insomnia represents a break from nature, and the degree to which the problem is pandemic suggests a societal dislocation of massive proportions. Insomniacs and sleep scientists alike, therefore, must constantly ask themselves how we can reestablish a symbiotic bond with the natural forces of the cosmos. As individuals and as a society, we must try to heal our break with nature and live once again in harmony with our environment. When we do that, we will all sleep better.

Getting Your Children to Sleep

There never was a child so lovely, but his mother was glad to get him to sleep.

RALPH WALDO EMERSON

*I*f you are a parent, you have at least two good reasons to make sure your child sleeps well: the child and you. The advantages of sound sleep for the health of your offspring should be obvious. As for yourself, a child who can't get to sleep can upset a parent's own pre-sleep routine, and a child who awakens in the night can knock adult sleep patterns out of kilter. In either case, parents might stay up nights worrying about what is wrong with the child.

In the first few months of life, infant sleep patterns vary enormously, and frequent awakenings are normal. After about three months, 70 percent of babies sleep through the night without interruption; by six months that number grows to about 83 percent. Approximately 10 percent do not establish a pattern of sleeping through the night for more than a year (and some who do establish such a pattern early can revert to nighttime awakenings later on).

If after six months your child does not regularly settle down for the night, you should take a close look at his or her bedtime routine; you may have to make some changes to help the child get into healthy sleep habits. Dr. Richard Ferber, author of *Solve Your Child's Sleep Problems,* says, "If your routine is working, if you and your child are happy with it, if he falls asleep easily and night wakings are infrequent, if he is getting enough sleep and if his daytime behavior is appropriate, then it's likely that whatever is being done is fine." However, Dr. Ferber believes that some pre-sleep routines are more amenable to healthy nights than others.

One ritual he warns against is rocking your child to sleep at bedtime and again whenever the child awakens in the night. By doing this you might actually interfere with natural sleep and postpone the day when the child will sleep without interruption. A child who is always nursed or rocked to sleep might have trouble going back to sleep on her own after nighttime arousals, which are normal. Hence, in many cases, it is important to put the child down while she is still awake so she can learn to settle into sleep on her own.

Another routine Dr. Ferber warns against is allowing your child to share your bed. Even if you and your spouse don't object, and even if the child seems to sleep well in your bed, making a habit of it can be detrimental for both the parents and the child. "Although taking your child into bed with you for a night or two may be reasonable if he is ill or very upset about something," says Dr. Ferber, "for the most part this is not a good idea. We know for a fact that people sleep better alone in bed." Sleeping better is only one reason for having your child sleep alone; it is also important for him to learn how to separate from you without anxiety and to see himself as an independent individual. Dr. Ferber's recommendation to let children sleep alone pertains to single parents as well. For one thing, a child who can't sleep alone is hard to leave with a sitter. More important, the child might already feel responsible for the parents' separation; sleeping with the remaining parent might reinforce this burdensome, albeit erroneous, belief.

It should be emphasized that an opposing point of view to Dr. Ferber's exists, and that many parents feel their young children *should* share the parental bed at night. In an important book, *The Family Bed*, Tine Thevenin makes a strong argument in favor of parents and babies sleeping together. She points out that separate sleeping rooms constitute a relatively new phenomenon found predominantly in the Western world. A counselor for the La Leche League, Thevenin believes that sharing the parental bed is a way to solve a child's sleep problems and create a closer bond between family members. She contends that if a parent takes his or her child into the parental bed instead of letting the child cry to sleep, the child will have a stronger sense of security. Thevenin backs up her views with endorsements from parents and from authorities such as anthropologist Ashley Montague.

Inconsistency is another factor that can destroy a child's peaceful slumber. A reasonable and consistent structure of feeding, playing, bathing, and other regular activities will help his system stabilize a sleep/wake rhythm. Dr. Ferber urges parents to establish regular routines in the first three months of life. "Your child cannot be expected to keep to a schedule on his own," he writes; "you will have to set a reasonable one for him and then be willing to enforce it."

Regular routines are important throughout childhood and into adolescence. Many experts recommend that you not let your toddler decide what time he or she should go to bed. Such permissiveness invariably leads to haphazard schedules that carry over to eating, playing, and other activities and can create disorder. At the same time, parents should be flexible and respect the natural differences among children. Don't base your child's routine entirely on your personal convenience, but adapt to the cues offered by the child's physiology and behavior.

THE BEDTIME ROUTINE

Perhaps the most important factor in establishing a routine is to be sure the time preceding sleep is pleasant so the child looks forward to it instead of resenting it. The routine should be followed every night as consistently as possible, and in it one or both parents should spend time with the child. Tell or show your child the sequence: for example, changing into pajamas, reading a story, and saying good-night to siblings. Tell your child exactly what bedtime activities have been planned and how much time will be spent on them. Let him or her know you will not extend the pre-sleep period beyond the agreed-upon limit.

Experts also advise setting aside 10 to 30 minutes right before bed to do something special with your child. Keep in mind that bedtime means separation, and for many children that can be a difficult adjustment. Avoid scary stories, teasing, or anything that will excite the child. Quiet play, story reading, and discussion of school, family events, future activities, and similar subjects are recommended. The atmosphere should be close, warm, and personal—watching TV together will not suffice.

For young children, a special toy or blanket might be part of the bedtime ritual. Called "transitional objects," these inanimate sleep companions can help the child accept nighttime separation by providing comfort and reassurance in your absence. The doll, toy, blanket, or stuffed animal might give the child a feeling of control over her world.

Many children select a transitional object in their toddler years and stick with it loyally. If you notice that your child favors a particular doll or toy, you might include it in the bedtime ritual by having it "listen in" to the storytelling or tucking it in with your child. If your child does not have a favorite toy, many pediatricians suggest offering her one that you think is a good choice, bearing in mind not to force the selection on the child.

When a child reaches age nine or ten, she typically begins to want privacy before bed. Honor this need, but it is still advisable to drop in for a short chat and a loving good-night.

IF YOUR CHILD HAS TROUBLE SLEEPING

Children can be insomniacs too, and usually their sleep problems are psychologically based. Although kids can certainly get sad or forlorn, they seldom display the classic symptoms of depression before puberty. However, young children are no strangers to other sleep-robbing emotions—they worry, they get angry, they feel rejected (as when a new sibling comes along and usurps parental attention), they get scared.

Some children develop anxieties directly related to sleeptime. "From infancy on, many children associate going to sleep with leaving the world behind," wrote Dr. Ira L. Mintz in *Parents' Magazine*. "The leaving is synonymous with separating from the mother, since the mother . . . provides the warmth, food, affection and love necessary for life." Fearful of this separation, the child might find excuses of all kinds to postpone bed and then have difficulty falling asleep or returning to sleep after waking up during the night. Dr. Mintz suggests developing trust by instituting brief separations each day. Times apart demonstrate to the child that he is still safe even though you are absent, and they reassure him that his parents will be there again when a brief separation ends.

Night terrors can also generate a fear of falling asleep. A child who encounters monsters in the night will, understandably, not look forward to closing his eyes the next night. If your child has had an unsettling nightmare, get him to talk about his experience, suggests Los Angeles psychiatrist Mark Goulston. You should act as a shock absorber. Try not to get impatient and don't dismiss the experience by saying, "It was only a dream."

A good way to help your child purge the nightmare is to

ask a question such as "How scared are you?" This tells the child you are not going to gloss over her experience; you are going to listen. "What do you remember?" is another evocative question, and it can be followed by specific questions about the dream itself. Responses such as "That never happens during the day, but it's a heck of a dream" and "I hated scary dreams like that when I was your age" are also reassuring. "What you want to do is milk the terror out of the child," says Dr. Goulston.

Of course, it is not only sleep-related anxieties that keep a child awake. When a child is anxious it is usually because he feels overwhelmed by, for example, a certain change in his life that he is not prepared to handle. It is important to get the child to express his fears. "If you can communicate to the child that you know how he feels," says Dr. Goulston, "this will often put the anxiety to rest. Nothing is more comforting to a child than knowing that his parents understand how he feels and that they are minding the store."

Dr. Goulston also points out that a child gets his sense of well-being from how his parents relate to each other. The child needs to feel that his parents love each other and are happy together. Studies have shown that children often pick up on unresolved conflicts in the family. Any sign of dissension and conflict can keep a child awake, terrified that his security is being torn asunder. Therefore, says Goulston, if your child is having sleep problems due to anxiety, look to yourself and your marriage. Try to increase your awareness of family dynamics and with or without the help of a therapist work out any unresolved conflicts. Your child will sleep a lot better if you do—and so will you.

Bibliography

Bauer, W., *All You Need to Know about Insomnia, Sleep and Dreams* (New York: Essandes, 1967).

Bieler, Henry, *Food is Your Best Medicine* (New York: Random House, 1965).

Buhler, W., *How to Overcome Sleeplessness* (Los Angeles: Krishna Press, 1973).

Ceres, *Herbs to Help You Sleep* (England: Thorsens Publishers, 1972).

Consumer Reports, *Drug Information for the Consumer* (Mt. Vernon, N.Y.: Consumer Reports Books, 1987).

Crisp, Arthur, *Sleep, Nutrition and Mood* (New York: Stonehill, 1976).

Dement, William, *Some Must Watch While Some Must Sleep* (New York: W. H. Freeman, 1974).

Dintenfass, Julius, *Chiropractic: A Modern Way to Health* (New York: Pyramid, 1970).

Dryer, Bernard, *Inside Insomnia* (New York: Random House, 1986).

Dufty, William, *Sugar Blues* (New York: Warner, 1976).

Duncan, A. H., *Everything You Want to Know about Sleep* (New York: Pyramid, 1973).

Ferber, Richard, *Solve Your Child's Sleep Problems* (New York: Simon and Schuster, 1985).

Foulkes, Davis, *The Psychology of Sleep* (New York: Scribner's, 1966).

Hartmann, Ernest L., *The Functions of Sleep* (New Haven: Yale Press, 1973).

_____ . *The Sleeping Pill* (New Haven: Yale University Press, 1978).

_____ . *The Sleep Book* (New York: American Association of Retired People, 1987).

Kales, Anthony, *Sleep: Physiology and Pathology* (Philadelphia: Lippincott, 1969).

Kelly, Charles, *The Natural Way to Healthful Sleep* (New York: Hawthorne, 1961).

Kleitman, Nathaniel, *Sleep and Wakefulness* (Chicago: University of Chicago, 1963).

Kohler, M., and Chapelle, J., *101 Recipes for Sound Sleep* (New York: Funk and Wagnalls, 1967).

Kovel, Joel, *The Complete Guide to Therapy: From Psychoanalysis to Behavior Modification* (New York: Pantheon, 1977).

Linde, Shirley, *The Sleep Book* (New York: Harper and Row, 1974).

Luce, Gay, and Segal, J., *Sleep* (New York: Coward-McCann, 1966).

_____ . *Insomnia: The Guide for Troubled Sleepers* (New York: Doubleday, 1969).

Meares, A., *Relief without Drugs* (New York: Doubleday, 1965).

Phillips, Elliot, *Get a Good Night's Sleep* (New York: Prentice Hall, 1983).

Regestein, Quentin, *Sound Sleep* (New York: Simon and Schuster, 1980).

Rubenstein, Hillary, *Insomniacs of the World, Goodnight!* (New York: Random House, 1974).

Samuels, Mike, *The Well Body Book* (New York: Random House, 1973).

Scott, Cyril, *Good Sleep without Drugs* (New York: Lust, 1974).

Selye, Hans, *The Stress of Life* (New York: McGraw-Hill, 1956).

Slagle, Priscilla, *The Way Up from Down* (New York: Random House, 1987).

Steincrohn, Peter, *How to Get a Good Night's Sleep* (Chicago: Regnery, 1968).

Sussman, J., *How to Sleep without Drugs* (New York: Hippocrene Books, 1986).

Sweeney, Donald, *Overcoming Insomnia: A Medical Program for Problem Sleepers* (New York: Putnam, 1989).

Thevenin, Tine, *The Family Bed* (Garden City Park, N.Y.: Avery Publishing, 1987).

Thoresen, Carl, and Coates, T., *How to Sleep Better* (Englewood Cliffs, N.J.: Prentice Hall, 1976).

Webb, Wilse, *Sleep: The Gentle Tyrant* (New York: Spectrum, 1975).

Weitzman, Elliot, *Advances in Sleep Research Volumes I and II* (New York: Halsted Press, 1974, 1976).

Index

About the Authors

Philip Goldberg is a professional writer specializing in psychology and medicine. The author of 10 nonfiction books, including *The Intuitive Edge* and *The Babinski Reflex*, he is also a screenwriter and novelist. He and his wife Jane currently sleep in Los Angeles.

Daniel Kaufman is a Fulbright scholar, professional writer, passionate painter, and literary agent. He lives by the sea with his wife Gina and daughter Anastasia.